At the Foot of Dragon Hill

At the Foot of Dragon Hill

Florence J. Murray, M.D.

E.P. DUTTON & COMPANY, INC. | NEW YORK | 1975

LIBRARY OF CONGRESS CATALOGING IN PUBLICATION DATA
Murray, Florence J 1894–
At the foot of Dragon Hill.

1. Murray, Florence J., 1894– 2. Missionaries, Medical—Korea—Correspondence, reminiscences, etc. 3. Women physicians—Correspondence, reminiscences, etc. I. Title.
R722.M8 1975 266'.025'0924 [B] 75–14424

First Edition

10 9 8 7 6 5 4 3 2 1

Published simultaneously in Canada by Clarke, Irwin & Company Limited, Toronto and Vancouver
ISBN: 0–525–05991–1

To
the memory of
my father and mother who always encouraged me

Preface

I admit to making my first appearance at my maternal grandmother's home in Pictou Landing, a village on Nova Scotia's north shore, on a stormy February day in 1894. The next year, my brother Alexander was born. At the time my father was a theological student at Pine Hill Divinity Hall, a Presbyterian theological college. Mother had been a schoolteacher.

Their home was at West River, and there I spent my first two years. I loved my baby brother so much I wanted to give him things, including sticks of firewood put on top of him in his cradle.

After graduation Father took a congregation at Lawrencetown near Halifax, where my second brother was born. I have little recollection of that period, but Mother told me later that I had once seized a piece of wood and drove away a big boy who had ventured to touch my little brother.

When I was six, Father moved the family to a new congregation at Earltown village where we lived for ten years. There two brothers, Edward and Charles, and a sister Anna, were born. We older ones attended the one-room, ten-grade school.

Growing up in a farming community, the only careers that

I knew of open to girls were teaching, nursing, and stenography, none of which appealed to me. I wanted to do something different.

When I told my parents I would like to be a minister, Father, although doubtful of the possibility, accompanied me to the church headquarters for Eastern Canada at Halifax. The official there was sympathetic but told me kindly that the Presbyterian Church wasn't yet ready to accept women ministers.

I then decided to be a doctor. Father and Mother thought this possible and said they would do all they could to help me achieve my desire. According to today's standards, on Father's salary of 750 dollars annually, we were in dire poverty, but we never even suspected it. We had all we needed and as much as our neighbors had. We made our own playthings and fun, and life was good. To save money for our education Mother made our clothes and was economical in everything, often going without things she should have had for herself.

My father had hoped to go abroad as a missionary with three of his classmates at Pine Hill. I believe he applied to go, but the church budget at the time was sufficient for only three. Father, having a wife and child would need more to live on than single men who therefore got the appointments and became the founders of the Canadian Presbyterian Mission in Korea.

When these missionaries came home on furlough, they visited Father, and I was fascinated by their stories of life and conditions in Korea. Dr. Robert Grierson had trained a staff and ran a hospital and I thought what he was doing was wonderful. Dr. Kate MacMillan also treated patients in a two-room mud house, but was hoping for a better building soon. I decided I would go and help in my father's place.

Father's next pastorate was in Prince Edward Island where Alexander and I attended Prince of Wales College in Charlottetown.

While there, students from our college returned from a quadrennial North American student volunteer conference in Nashville. They gave enthusiastic reports and made earnest appeals for students to volunteer for overseas work: teaching, preaching, and healing.

Alex and I each decided to go. Neither of us told the other, but we both wrote to our parents, who informed me then that at my birth they had dedicated me to the Lord and were happy that I had made such a decision.

On passing the matriculation examination, I was accepted at Dalhousie University Medical College in Halifax. Sometime later, I discovered that McGill and other well-known universities were still refusing to accept women in medicine. Years before, Dalhousie had begun to accept the first qualified women who applied, and now had numerous women graduates.

The principal of Prince of Wales College and various others tried to discourage me, saying that instructors and students would hate having a woman in the class and would make it unpleasant for me. Yet, never once in my five years in medical school did I encounter any unpleasantness. My classmates were gentlemen and by the end of our course were almost like brothers.

I entered medical college in 1914, the year the first great war started in Europe. Instructors and students soon began dropping out of university to join the armed forces, and finally only ten remained in my class.

We students all felt that since our brothers, cousins, and classmates were fighting and dying in the trenches in France, this was no time for dances or other fun. We indulged in walking parties and an occasional movie, but most spare time was given to Red Cross work, making and folding dressings and bandages and preparing and sending socks, food, and chocolate to the boys overseas.

Alex's artillery unit was also due to ship out, but the time of departure was a military secret and I never had a chance to say goodbye. Foster, however, was training in a signal corps near Halifax and we got to see each other often.

On December 6, 1917, during my fourth year, there occurred the greatest man-made explosion in history up to that time. A French munitions ship loaded with TNT collided with a Belgian relief vessel and blew up in Halifax harbor. This explosion destroyed half the city, killed two thousand people and wounded ten thousand. No one will ever know how many more were washed into the harbor by the resulting tidal wave. All senior medical students rushed to help. The military set up emergency hospitals to care for the thousands of emergency cases. I reported for duty at the YMCA emergency hospital.

"Has your class had instruction in anesthesia?" asked the commanding officer. "Yes, sir," I replied. There was no opportunity to say that all in the class except myself had had this training. In the army one doesn't explain. One answers questions.

"Go to the operating room and give anesthetics," ordered the officer.

The first patient was six years old. Did a child require the same amount of anesthetic as an older person, or should she have a smaller dose? I didn't know. I knew I should watch the eye reflexes to help judge the depth of anesthesia, but this unfortunate child had lost both eyes. In fear and trembling, I gave that anesthetic and others following it all day. The next morning the commanding officer appointed me official anesthetist for the hospital.

In 1918, during my fifth year, the first worldwide epidemic of what came to be called Spanish flu struck the country. No one knew at first what it was, nor what could be done for it. There were many complications and hundreds died. At eleven o'clock one night the chief public health official for the province called me up.

"I want you to take the early train tomorrow to Lockport," he said. "Twenty-five people have died in that small fishing town and now the doctor has got the disease."

"I'd like to help," I said, "but I'm a student without medical equipment or license to practice."

"I know that, but the situation is desperate. So many doctors are overseas, there's no one else to send. Use the doctor's equipment, and phone me if you get into any trouble."

I took the morning train and found the situation *was* desperate. In some homes every person had influenza, and not one was able to prepare food for the others.

The community set up an emergency hospital in the public hall. I phoned for nurses. Two days later they arrived, two of them. One became the first patient as she had developed the sickness on the train and so went straight to the hospital.

One good citizen was heard to declare that he would have no petticoat doctor around him if he contracted the disease. He did, but by that time he had changed his mind about petticoat doctors.

The epidemic had reached its peak when I arrived and there were no more deaths. I did what I could, but probably received more credit than I earned.

Our studies were somewhat disrupted by so many of our instructors being in the services, but that was somewhat compensated for by the experience we gained treating victims of the explosion and the epidemic, and by assisting overworked specialists in surgery and obstetrics. However, the superintendant of the Victoria General Hospital, where most medical graduates got internships, was a businessman who had no use for women interns.

I not only wanted an internship, I wanted one of the few that paid a salary. I felt I had to repay as much as I could of what had been expended on my education. The first place I heard about that—in addition to room and board—paid the munificent salary of eleven dollars a week, was the Long Island Hospital in Boston Harbor. I applied and got on the staff as an intern.

I soon found that interns were left largely on their own with little in the way of supervision or instruction. Most patients were indigents, old friendless people, and unmarried pregnant girls referred to disparagingly by the men on the staff as soiled doves. A few of the medical staff were kind and sympathetic, but the general atmosphere was critical, and I was distressed at the low standard of medical care given and the lack of consideration for the feelings of the patients.

I once saw one of the staff doctors wash out the mouth of an old and weak diabetic patient with soap—childish and vengeful conduct. The old woman had been impertinent, not without provocation. I decided the Long Island Hospital was not for me.

Getting a weekend off, I returned to Halifax to consult with Dr. J. G. MacDougall, one of the chief surgeons in Nova Scotia, whom I had assisted throughout my final year. He offered me a position as his assistant. I could also hang out my shingle and take what patients came. I resigned from the Long Island Hospital. Soon, I also had a position as demonstrator of anatomy in the medical college.

When I had refunded a worthwhile amount into the family coffer, I informed the Mission Board of the Canadian Presbyterian Church that I was now ready to go overseas.

They had had a request from Dr. Kate MacMillan in Korea for a woman doctor to assist her. Would I go?

I would.

Friends wondered why I wanted to go so far away? Was I crazy? (Some still ask that.)

I went because Korea then had few trained doctors and more diseases than we in the West. Many people were without medical care, victims of ignorance, superstition, and fear of evil spirits alleged to cause disease. Dr. MacMillan had worked alone for years and needed help, and I was young, strong, well-trained, and no longer needed in Canada now that the war was over and the medical people in the forces had returned. Why shouldn't I go? It would be a great adventure.

Furthermore, brought up as I was, in an earnest Christian home and with a strong personal faith, I wanted to use my life where it would count most. I wanted to serve others and share my knowledge of God as our loving heavenly Father with people living in fear of evil spirits.

I went, and I've never regretted it.

I worked in Korea, with a furlough to the homeland every sixth year, until exchanged by the Japanese for their countrymen in America during World War II. That was 1942.

Canadian missionaries were finally permitted to return to Korea in 1947, but not to the North where we had lived and worked and which was now under communist control. I worked in the South till final retirement in 1969.

People sometimes ask me, "Were you a doctor or a missionary?" I hope I was both.

This is the story of my first two decades in Korea.

Florence J. Murray, M.D.
Pine Hill Drive
Halifax, N.S.

September 1974

At
the Foot
of Dragon Hill

-1-

A bull cart, accompanied by several anxious and exhausted people, drew up at the door of the mission hospital in Hamheung, Korea. The injured man in the cart was too far gone to speak. Dr. Kate MacMillan went out to see him, and I followed.

"My elder brother was gored by a bull three days ago," said the driver. "We've traveled ever since to get here and we haven't any money but do please help us. *Sal lyo chusio. Sal lyo chusio,"* he pleaded; literally, "give us his life, save him."

"Sal lyo chusio," begged the dying man's wife and mother, turning beseeching eyes on the foreign woman doctor, while the look of despair on the patient's face was more appealing than words.

"Let me see," said Dr. MacMillan, turning down the blood-stained quilt that covered the man.

Loops of intestine protruding through a gaping wound in the abdomen were black and gangrenous.

Gently the doctor said, "You'd better take him home. It's too late to save him." Stoically they turned away.

I was aghast. Surely the suffering man should be admitted, his passing made as easy as possible, and the weary travelers allowed to rest. Then I had my first lesson in the practice of medicine in Korea.

"If this man were to die in the hospital," said Dr. MacMillan, "his family would be terrified his spirit would haunt them. They'd prefer him to die on the road, as he certainly will, rather than in a strange place. If he could speak and understand the circumstances, he would insist on starting for home. Would he want his spirit, dying far from his native place, to roam restless forever? Besides, a death in the hospital means that other patients, fearful of his spirit haunting them, would refuse to stay. Seven hundred girls in the Yungsaing School across the way would hear the wailing for the dead and report in hundreds of homes that someone had died in the Cheihei Hospital. As a result, few would attend the clinic for days. It's better to continue treating those who can be helped."

Dr. MacMillan was a tall thin woman whose white hair and lined face made her look considerably older than her fifty-five years. More than twenty years of heavy work and responsibility carried almost alone, without even the bare minimum of equipment and facilities, had taken their toll. Worn and frail as she was, her alert blue eyes had a look of determination about them.

The mission hospital then consisted of several small boxlike rooms with two or three beds each on two floors.

The three-foot wide stairway had a right-angled turn which made it impossible to carry up a stretcher. If a patient couldn't walk, he had to be carried piggyback. The narrow corridors had no direct lighting. In the dimly lighted hallway where inpatient and outpatient areas met, I stumbled over an eight-inch-high step.

"This building was built from both ends," explained the doctor, "and when they met in the middle the floor levels didn't match. People often stumble, but nobody's ever been injured here."

In the operating room facing the south, the summer sun made the room extremely hot. The layer of concrete over the wooden floor was flaking off in great patches. Surgical instruments were scarce, out-of-date, and well worn.

Straw mattresses were hard and lumpy, sheets and blankets few; but that didn't matter, the doctor said, because patients preferred their own bedding and usually brought it with them. In government hospitals they had to provide their own and they expected the same here. Cracks in the wooden beds made fine lodging places for bedbugs that often came with the bedding. There was no running water, no bathtub, and no plumbing.

"How can you work under such conditions?" I asked.

"Coming from Canada no doubt you notice a difference," she replied. "Really, there's been much improvement. I used to live and work in a three-room Korean mud house. For several years there were no Korean doctors nor nurses. I had to train my assistants and for a long-time Kang Do-Ka [her long-time assistant and friend] was the only one I had. There was never money enough for proper equipment. But the church is supporting the medical work more now, and with you here we'll do great things together."

"It looks as though there's plenty to do," I said with a glance at the full waiting room.

"As for running water and baths, it doesn't matter as much as you think because patients are afraid of bathing when they're sick and if baths are insisted on, they are likely to go home. Since the attendants feel the same, everybody's satisfied as it is."

"No doubt it takes time to change old ideas."

"It does," said Kate MacMillan, "but they do change. One of the next things I want to work on is the laboratory. We must improve that."

In the outpatient dispensary, nursing attendants were busy in the two small examining and treatment rooms. Here I met Dr. Pak in a room crowded with patients.

"Look around by yourself now," said Kate MacMillan, "I must get to work."

Screen doors were propped open with chairs. People apparently felt more at home with flies and mosquitoes about. Later I learned that they didn't like beds, because they feared they would fall out of them and so preferred the floor for sleeping.

In the wards each patient had one or more—usually more—relatives with him. Sometimes the sick person was in the bed, sometimes someone else, sometimes two together. It was difficult to tell who was the patient. The family looked after the ill person in their own way, for they had little confidence in the nurses. If the doctor or hospital staff objected to what they did, they took the sick one home, often at night without the knowledge of doctor or cashier.

Outside the back door I was horrified to see a bedpan with its contents setting on the ground together with a pail of bloodstained dressings and a pan full of pus. All were swarming with flies. My heart sank. How could I ever maintain decent standards under such conditions? There would be plenty to do all right, but conditions must be improved. This would be a teaching job as well as a medical one.

The Presbyterian Church in Canada had appointed Annetta Rose, deaconess and teacher from Nova Scotia; Christina Currie, deaconess from Ontario; and me, medical doctor from Nova Scotia; as missionaries to Korea. We left our homes and traveled by train across the North American continent for nearly a week; for the first time, we saw the great prairies and mountains of our country. Sailing from Vancouver, British Columbia, by the Canadian Pacific liner *Empress of Japan,* we landed two weeks later at the Japanese port of Kobe.

In spite of the heat, we walked about the streets savoring the fascinating city. Among the multicolored and gaily patterned kimono-clad people, we were surprised to see on a back street by the river an entirely naked man strolling along. The sound of the wooden clogs, worn by nearly everybody, was so loud as to make conversation difficult. The smells of fish cooking mingled with that of sweat and sewers, together with several undiagnosed odors, were overpowering. This was the Orient. How could we react or adjust to it? Never had we seen such crowds of humanity.

A day on the train from Kobe to the port of Shimonoseki gave us a glimpse of country life: tiny mud farm houses, incredibly green rice fields, forest-clad mountains, and farmers and their wives wearing cone-shaped hats of straw bent in the fields. Their bronze faces seemed strange to us.

On boarding the ferry for Pusan, Korea, we found the few first- and second-class bunks occupied. The crowding in the third class, comprising the whole of the lower deck, was so great that there didn't seem to be space left for one more person to stretch out on the straw matting covering the floor. About three hundred men, women, and children were settling down among their luggage for the night. One look and one whiff was enough for us. We fled to the open deck where there was space and fresh air. The deck planks weren't much harder than the straw matting, and the stars overhead formed a comforting canopy.

At dawn, on September 1, 1921, we reached Pusan Harbor. Such was our eagerness that we were the first to go ashore. Having passed customs and immigration in Japan, we had only to change some money to Korean currency and obtain tickets for the express to Seoul. As most Korean passengers were buying third-class tickets, we bought them too.

The train was so crowded that we had to step over baggage piled in the aisles, and many had to stand for the entire twelve-hour trip to the capital. Yet, people seemed friendly and we felt helpless in not being able to reply to their questions. When the "boy" came through the car with Korean food in paper-thin wooden boxes, we each bought one and had our first experience with rice and chopsticks. Small earthenware pots of steaming Japanese tea were also for sale and proved quite refreshing.

As the train sped among pine-clad mountains, the deep green of the rice paddies began to show a touch of gold. White-robed farmers, with black horsehair hats and long bamboo pipes in their mouths, carried great loads on wooden frames on their backs. Women, also in white, wore short wide-sleeved jackets and pleated skirts down to their ankles. In addition to the usual baby on their backs, they carried loads on their heads, while trudging the narrow poplar-lined roads. Though the men bent under their burdens, the women were straight and erect as they strode along. Children in gay colors raced along the low dikes between the patchwork quilt of tiny rice fields.

The villages' brown mud houses and gray thatched roofs, clustered at the foot of the hills, looked like mushrooms. The narrow valleys and mountain slopes were terraced with level after level of rice paddies. Even the dikes between them were utilized for growing food, the darker green of soybeans forming miniature hedges. Not an inch was left unused.

Where the water caught the gleam of sunbeams between the rows of growing rice, it reflected them back like molten gold. Irrigation canals, bull carts, village after village in close proximity, dignified white-clad people, and swarms of children were everywhere.

Night fell before we entered the dimly lighted city of Seoul. At South Gate station, Edna Lawrence, a cheerful dark-haired nurse from Severance Mission Hospital met us. She gave our suitcases to a "jiggy" man who piled it on his carrying frame, squatted, and then thrust his arms through the straw shoulder ropes.

Korean laborers, I learned, had strong backs and preferred carrying loads on their jiggy frames to carrying them in their hands or pulling handcarts. Even a suitcase with a handle would be carried on the back. Rising easily to his feet under the burden, he followed as Edna led the way across the street into the Severance Hospital compound where we spent the night with Edna in the nurses' residence.

Another day going north on the train brought us late in the evening to our destination, the city of Hamheung. Ethel McEachran and Reverend Luther Young of the Canadian Presbyterian Mission met us at the station with one of the two cars in the province. The other belonged to the Japanese governor.

After a ride of about a mile through dark streets, Ethel and I got out on a narrow muddy path, while the others went on to the next mission house where the Robb family lived.

Taking my arm, Ethel guided me through a dark, crooked alley. Drains from several dwellings along the way crossed the path, but my companion was so familiar with it that she needed no light.

"Whatever's that smell?" I asked, stumbling along.

"Oh! Do you get a smell?" she said. "It's mostly drains and outhouses though they keep a pig in one yard. You'll soon get used to it."

Beyond a rickety wooden gate loomed a square boxlike wooden house, with a wide veranda.

"Welcome to the womens' house," said Ethel as she led me in. "I'm sorry I'm the only one to welcome you here, but Jennie Robb is on a country trip and won't be back for ten days and Dr. MacMillan has just been called to the hospital but should be back soon."

Ethel gave me a belated supper and then, with a candle, showed me upstairs to my room. She advised me to be careful tucking in the bottom of the mosquito net suspended over the bed.

"Tuck it in well under the mattress on all sides," she said, "for many of these mosquitoes buzzing around so hungrily are malaria carriers."

I followed her directions, and with thanks to God for the safe journey to my new home, I slept.

The sun rising over Dragon Hill next morning revealed a small room with two windows so high that all one could see on looking up at them was the edge of the roof tiles and a bit of sky. A series of low sliding panels ran along the back of the room and opened into a storage space so low that one couldn't stand up in it. Though the mud walls and ceiling of the house were nicely whitewashed, this failed to mute the musty smell of mud and straw that pervaded the place.

A further disadvantage of mud as a building material appeared one morning after someone had left a tap in the bathroom not quite turned off. The ceiling of the room beneath lay, in a highly viscous state, partly on the dining table, partly on the floor.

"Take the morning off," said Ethel at breakfast. "Mr. McCaul is here from Wonsan and he's going to show you around. Climb Dragon Hill, take a look at the hospital, and this afternoon you'll start language study. Your teacher is a young man by the name of Ahn Sang-Chul. The surname comes first in Korea. You'll call him Ahn Sunsaing, literally 'Ahn Before Born,' meaning Teacher Ahn. He'll be here at two o'clock."

The womens' house was surrounded by a mud wall topped with tiles. Over the wall I saw the thatched mud houses of our neighbors. There were similar houses inside the compound too—one for the "outside man," another for the cook and her household. Other houses from which the partitions had been removed served as classrooms for the primary department of the school.

The high school was a rectangular two-story building of such flimsy construction that the weight of the tile roof had caused the walls to bulge. They were kept relatively near their original position by metal bars running the length and width of the building, while the heavy tiles had been replaced by lighter corrugated iron. Ethel McEachran was the principal of both sections of the Yungsaing Girls' School.

On rising ground across a little gully stood the mission hospital: a two-story, red brick building with a sagging wood veranda in front.

Gordon McCaul took the three of us new arrivals up Dragon Hill back of the mission houses to show us the view. On the lower slopes were hundreds and hundreds of rounded mounds about six feet in diameter and three in height. This was the public cemetery for untold generations. Through and beyond this ancient graveyard a path led with many ups and downs along the top of the ridge. This suggested to the people of olden days the undulations on the back of a dragon, and hence the mountain's name.

From the summit, one got a fine view of the city and the surrounding countryside.

"Hamheung is one of the six largest cities in Korea," Mr. McCaul told us. "About 50,000 people live here."

Except for a few two-story buildings along the main streets, most construction consisted of one-story earthen houses. The well-to-do had tile roofs, the rest straw thatch. Street signs were in Chinese characters. There was no paving and no street lighting. Wind raised dust in clouds. In residential areas the streets were lined with mud walls. Wooden gates opened into courtyards which could not be seen from the street. Windows of paper admitted some light, but excluded curious stares of passersby.

West of the mission houses meandered an insignificant looking stream, all but lost in a wide expanse of sand.

"Not much of a river," Annetta remarked.

"Just wait till you see it in the rainy season," said McCaul. "It becomes a roaring torrent filling the whole area between those embankments. The rice plain beyond is the third largest in all Korea."

Little villages dotted the plain, brown thatched roofs peeking out from poplars and sycamores surrounding them. Blue in the distance, a range of mountains blended into the horizon.

Returning through the city, we were followed by crowds of children, their sparkling dark eyes fixed on the queer looking foreigners. *"Ma Moksa! Ma Moksa!"* they shouted looking at Mr. McCaul. *"Maing Pouine!"* they said looking at us. Gordon McCaul explained.

"Mr. McRae was the first foreigner to live here and his Korean name is *Ma Moksa,* meaning pastor. So *Ma Moksa* is Pastor McRae, but to these children it just means foreign man. *Maing* is Dr. MacMillan's Korean name, and *pouine* is a polite word for woman; so they are saying you are foreign women."

That first afternoon I began a long struggle with the difficult Korean language. Our teacher, Ahn Sunsaing, was of medium height, modest and kindly, conscientious, eager to do his best to guide my faltering tongue. He wore the national dress—a short white jacket, baggy white trousers tied neatly at the ankles with narrow blue ribbon, topped by a long white robe fastened in front by a one-loop knot, and white rubber shoes that he left on the doorstep.

"Ahn yung ha simnika?" "Are you in peace?" He greeted me each morning with a deep bow.

"Ahn yung ha simnika?" I replied, returning the bow. I repeated this many times till he was satisfied. He was patient, but the going was hard and sometimes I looked at him almost in despair. He encouraged me by telling me I was doing fine. It takes much time and practice to get our tongues around Korean sounds not found in English. And so, for some weeks, life consisted of struggles with the language, walks on Dragon Hill, and visits to the hospital.

Besides Dr. MacMillan, the medical staff in 1921 consisted of Dr. Pak, a young graduate of one of the recently started medical schools. Several girls and youths, being given some training by the doctors, served as nursing attendants. An elderly woman, Dr. MacMillan's long-time friend and assistant, was matron of the dormitory and general factotum of the hospital. Her name was Kang Do-Ka or Dorcas Kang.

The nursing attendants took temperatures, changed dressings, and gave injections, without which no patient considered he was getting any worthwhile treatment. I was amazed at the number of infected sores, abscesses, and wounds and shocked at the poor technique used in the treatment room of the dispensary. On finding family attendants and visitors removing dressings with their fingers to see how the wound was progressing, I began to see how the staff could easily realize their own technique hardly mattered.

Their supervisor, Kang Do-Ka, was a tiny bright-eyed kindly woman about the doctor's own age. Her black hair, parted neatly in the middle, drawn smoothly back from her brow, and fastened in a bun at the nape of her neck by a single silver pin, was showing streaks of white. This entitled her to be called grandmother by young people. She dressed in white as befitted an elderly woman, but was still as active and energetic as any of the young folk. Quite devoted to Dr.

MacMillan, she felt as much responsible for what went on in the hospital as the doctor herself.

Though married women in Korea may change their given names, they don't take their husband's family name but retain their own. On account of high infant mortality, people considered it hardly worthwhile to name a baby until they were sure it was going to live. Even then, in Do-Ka's youth, girls often weren't given names at all. They were known merely as Teacher Kang's second daughter, or Carpenter Pak's girl child. *Tui-pangie,* literally "Back Room," meaning "born in the back room," and *Sup-suppie,* "Sorrow," expressing disappointment that a girl was born instead of a son, were common names for girls.

Under the Japanese rule, everyone had to be registered and names became necessary. If his women folk lacked names, the head of the household had to provide them. Yet, he might not think it important enough to inform the women what their impromptu official names were. So in my early days in the country I often had women patients who didn't know their own names and some who denied having any.

Until they had sons, their husbands called them *"Yopo"* or "Hi, you." Upon attaining motherhood, they were known as Baby's Mother. I once heard a list of names read out in church to which the pastor added, "In case anyone doesn't know her name, So-and-So is Elder Song's wife, So-and-So is Deacon Pak's wife, and So-and-So is the wife of Elder Lee." Another time So-and-So was announced as Elder Han's wife, and Such-a-One as Deacon Song's spouse.

Boys were sometimes given such names as Calf or even Dog Dung to deceive the spirits into thinking the child wasn't valued. Otherwise, the spirits might take revenge on the parents for any fancied neglect by causing sickness in the child.

When nameless women became Christians, they often chose names for themselves from the Bible. Whether Kang Do-Ka chose her name for herself, or the doctor chose it for her, it suited her well. For like her Biblical namesake, Dorcas, she was always doing something for others.

Nursing, however, was not considered a respectable job. For a young woman to nurse someone of another family, especially a man, was almost unthinkable. Therefore, few families would permit a daughter to do any sort of work in a hospital. Besides marriage, which was inevitable, the only acceptable positions for girls were as a teacher or a "maid-of-all-work" in a household. Though schools of nursing had been established in a few mission and government hospitals, it was difficult to get girls with any education to train.

Cooking for patients was done by their families: outdoors in summer, in the corridor or ward in winter. Their braziers left many burnt patches on the floors.

The doctors seemed to work in great confusion with whole families coming in the examining room, the eldest describing the patient's symptoms in detail, others breaking in from time to time with their observations. The patient, if a woman, would not be allowed to reply to the doctor's questions. What did she know, compared to a man?

On asking if this confusion were necessary, I was assured it was. The sick person wouldn't come to the hospital without the moral support of the family, nor would the family think of such a thing. However, confidence was increasing.

Dr. MacMillan sometimes asked me what I would do in certain circumstances, but my ideas were not usually practicable. Either she had already tried what I suggested and it hadn't worked or she was sure such a course of action would never be accepted by the Koreans.

Obviously, there was much to learn besides what was taught in medical school. The doctor seemed to know how best to handle any situation and I was eager to get to work, but it was necessary to learn Korean before I could work effectively. So I had to leave her and young Dr. Pak to struggle on by themselves while I went to language school in Seoul.

-2-

We three newcomers—Annetta Rose, who preferred to be called Rosie, Christina Currie, and I—together with Reverend Reg and Flossie McMullin of our mission, and about twenty others from sister missions, studied at the Seoul language school for six weeks. The mornings were spent with private tutors, the afternoons in class where Korean teachers taught us to understand and speak Korean and older missionaries explained the grammar.

In shops and marketplaces, we tried out our speaking ability on long-suffering, patient people. We often competed to see who could bargain for and buy the largest number of articles with fifty sen, about twenty-five cents. It was possible, we found, to buy six or seven brush pens, a stick of solid ink, a pair of bamboo chopsticks, a paper fan, an envelope, a postage stamp, and a cloth thimble or reel for winding thread.

The Korean alphabet is said to be the most scientific in the world. Its twenty-four letters expressed phonetically every sound in the language, but unfortunately the sounds weren't quite the same as in English. Though spelling was simple and went according to rule, with neither capital letters nor punctuation to bother about, it looked strangely foreign when written, since it read from right to left vertically instead of horizontally. Unfortunately for foreigners attempting to learn it, many Chinese characters were also used and they were neither few nor simple. That first term, we were expected to master only one hundred of them.

The Korean alphabet was simple enough so that on Sunday we could sing with the congregation even though we didn't understand the words. It was good to join in church life even to that extent.

Learning that Korean history went back four thousand years, we wondered where *our* ancestors were then and when *their* history began. We found that peace-loving Korea, though often having to defend herself, had never fought a war of aggression. We were surprised to hear that two hundred years before movable type had been thought of in Europe, Koreans had invented and used it. Also, the first encyclopedia in the world was written and published in Korea. A thousand years ago, Korean ceramics were famous throughout the Orient for grace and color. And back in the sixteenth century, a Korean admiral built the world's first armor-clad ships with which he defeated the greatest Japanese warrior in history.

With all respect for the past, our task was to learn present-day Korean as quickly as we could. It took time. One difficulty was to know the proper degree of respect to use in addressing various persons. Older people and those in high social standing had to be spoken to in special terms, but to use the same words to children or servants was to make oneself ridiculous.

I resolved to try it myself one day when Ahn Sunsaing answered my telephone call.

"Noo goo?" I heard him say. (Who is it?) *"Noo goo yo? Noo goo sio? Noo goo simnika? Noo goo onika?"*

My gracious, I thought, answering the phone wasn't yet for me.

When no reply came Ahn asked again using a slightly higher form. He might have gone as far down the scale as he went up. Using "low talk" to someone who merits more respect gives offense, while "high talk" to a child or much younger person is absurd. To judge the age or social position of everyone was a delicate business, and, in order to avoid the possibility of giving offense, we language students tried to use moderately high talk to all but children. Eventually we learned to be more selective.

At this time, Christina, Edith Kerr from Australia, and I were boarding with the Billings family, Methodist missionaries from the United States. On their Thanksgiving Day, they invited us to a masquerade party. We went as missionaries on furlough, looking as queer and old-fashioned as missionaries were popularly supposed to be. Dressed in our hostess's cast-off clothing, my hair up, and wearing a mask, I looked as funny as Christina who was attired in a long dress with a collar up to her ears and a tiny hat perched on the top of her head.

I had to represent my side in a contest to see who could talk longest without stopping for breath. Thinking I might talk longer if I didn't have to think what to say, I told the story of the rat that went into a granary and carried out one grain of wheat and another and another and another, and I won easily. For refreshments, we had delicious Korean apples and popcorn. Thus missionaries, on occasion, had a good time without a hangover.

One day, a boy from our own mission area came to the door looking for work. He had come to Seoul with more faith than funds to study. When his money gave out he tried to sell patent medicines on the streets, but there was little sale for his goods and when he came to the Billings' home he hadn't eaten for two days. We helped him temporarily and Mr. Billings made some inquiries about a job for him without avail. It was difficult for students to earn their way as the pay for anything they could get to do was so small. It was a common dilemma. Christina's teacher, Ahn Sunsaing, had dropped out of college for lack of money. He wished to study medicine, but hadn't the means.

At examination time, word came from our northern station, Yongjung, across the border in Manchuria, that Dr. Martin had been ill in bed for more than ten weeks. The clinic was falling off and they wanted me to come as soon as possible. The Martins were to go on furlough when the doctor was able to travel and I should be getting ready to take over. They wanted me to do some shopping for them as there wasn't much to buy in Yongjung and no one wished to undertake the long tiresome trip to Seoul unless it was necessary.

At the Seoul railway station, after answering all the questions of the police, we tried to get our luggage aboard the train amid great confusion and no haste. With train time approaching and our stuff still on the platform, Mr. McMullin, in not too fluent Korean, asked for action.

"Don't excite!" replied the baggage master with equal fluency. And indeed, there was no need. Somehow at the very last minute, in true Oriental fashion, the baggage got aboard and we were off. A fussing, fuming foreigner with a big nose is, to a Korean, a comical sight. Why wear oneself out all for a few minutes of time? Why indeed?

-3-

At Hamheung, we all reported as usual to the police at the railway station and, again as usual, those gentlemen arrived at our houses next morning at breakfast time to ask the same questions once more.

Miss Rose had been appointed to Hoiryung station where the McMullins lived and I to Yongjung farther on, so we and the McMullins were all to travel together. Ahn Sunsaing hadn't been able to get his passport in time to go with us.

Since the McMullins were guests and Rosie and I were to leave so soon, there was a round of gaiety to speed us on our way. The McMullins and I went to tea at the Robbs, Rosie and the McMullins came to supper at our house and Ethel would have invited the whole town only there weren't enough dishes.

Rosie and I were moving so we had to pack everything we had in Hamheung. When at last we got off, three jiggy men carried our luggage. At the railway station each had to be paid separately, everything weighed, and excess baggage charges paid, platform passes bought to let the men through the wicket with our belongings, and our train tickets bought. Then the jiggy men demanded even more money. Each transaction took so long that by the time we had told the police our names, ages, destinations, how long we were going to stay, and why we were going our patience was nearly gone. We knew we might be asked for our passports at any time and our luggage was subject to inspection whenever the customs officials felt curious. The departing bell rang, and we rushed on board to shouts from the carriers demanding more money.

To go north we first had to go south to the port of Wonsan where our freight from Canada was waiting. We found some had to be repacked for the rough trip ahead, since trunks and boxes were simply dropped into the hold and anything might be dumped on top of them.

After a look at the mission school for girls—a fine new brick building—the boys' school, and the Bible Institute where the Misses McCully trained women church workers, we sent our heavy goods off on carts to the wharf. Jiggy men took the hand baggage on their carrying frames, and we had walked a mile on the way to the pier when we met Gordon McCaul coming to tell us the ship's departure was delayed till the next afternoon. Back we went to the mission for the night.

Next day at the pier, we climbed down into sampans together with the baggage and crowds of Koreans and Japanese standing as close as they could pack in and were rowed out to the ship anchored in midharbor.

Sampans are flat-bottomed craft with square sterns in which a standing man steers and propels the boat with a long, curved oar. Bigger sampans towed by small ones took the freight.

The *Tategami Maru* plying from Japanese ports along the east coast to Vladivostock was the biggest and best ship on the route. We were fortunate to get first-class cabins with clean berths. Second-class passengers slept, men and women together, on the lower deck. Third class was poorer still, but since accommodation was limited, that was often all that was available. A Japanese meal was served, but the smell of the ship, a mingling of fish, hot grease, and sweat, failed to tempt us and we were glad we had brought our own food.

We arrived at the port of Sungjin next morning at five and

went ashore for the day. A walk of a mile and a half took us to the mission houses where Maud Rogers, principal of the mission girls' school welcomed us.

The Ross family invited us to breakfast. Their two small daughters played with their dolls tied to their backs in the way that Korean mothers carried their babies and they spoke Korean better than English. When the older child spoke in Korean to Miss Rogers, Maud asked her why she spoke Korean to her. "Jeannie English no can speak," replied the four year old.

That evening we boarded the *Tategami* again, but this time the sea was rough and we had to watch the waves as they rolled in as we leaped from the sampan to the gangway on the side of the ship between them. Rosie misjudged her timing and a wave caught her on the lower step. She scrambled up dripping to the knees.

At Chungjin next morning, we had to jump from the gangway to the sampan exactly when a wave brought it close. If we moved too late, we would end up in the harbor between ship and boat.

Our party had no trouble with customs inspection though Koreans had to open everything, have their pockets searched, and show the inside of their purses—all in their own country.

We utilized an eight-hour wait for the train to Hoiryung by buying more straw rope and again tying up our baggage so carefully packed at Wonsan. One box even had to be renailed. Then we piled everything on the flat car of a dinky little railroad, the rails about eighteen inches apart, to go the mile and a half to the "big" railway station. A man running behind with a long stick pushed the car till he got it going well. Then he leaped on and coasted till it began to slow down. Then he repeated the process. It was fun, but cold riding in the open.

The big train was also narrow gauge but wider. It ran along the Tuman River dividing Korea on its eastern side from Manchuria.

At Hoiryung, all three Canadian residents were at the station to welcome the McMullins back and to greet Rosie. Here, too, a mission school for girls had been recently built. The church people conducted the school for boys. Koreans built their own churches but, at that time, needed help with the schools. Government schools in the towns provided educational facilities for only about twenty percent of those eager to attend. Unless mission or church provided the means, most children of Christians would have had no opportunity whatever for an education. There was a Japanese hospital in Hoiryung, but no mission medical facility.

We telegraphed to Yongjung to announce my arrival. Telegrams could be sent from any post office and were not only quicker but more dependable than letters which frequently went astray. Telephones were few and far between.

The Hoiryung mission station was a bare, dreary place surrounded on three sides by Chinese gardens, chiefly characterized by the smell of human waste that was used as fertilizer. On the third side stood the city crematory whose odor did nothing to overcome the other smells. The missionary's wife said she had gotten used to it, but not to the nighttime howls of wild animals that she feared were wolves, hyenas, or tigers in the hills.

The high winds that blew almost constantly came right through the flimsily built houses. The walls were only one brick thick, plastered on the inside with mud, over which was a thin coat of plaster. Furnaces, just arrived from Canada and soon to be installed, gave hope of more comfort.

The couple's eleven-year-old had been lonely with his brother at school in Japan. His mother was teaching him at home that year. He had shot several pheasants that were delicious eating and had twice the meat of domesticated fowls.

I continued my journey next day by the same railway to its terminus at Sambong. Seats along the sides of the cars left plenty of standing space. Passengers did their own stoking of a smoky coal stove in the middle of the car and, when darkness fell, lighted the kerosene lamp in a bracket on the wall.

The Hoiryung mission secretary-evangelist, who had been suddenly deported from Manchuria without even a chance to bid goodbye to his wife and family, came with me as far as Sambong. He was sent out of the country because the Japanese there recognized him as a leader and, as such, regarded him with suspicion.

Amidst stolid Koreans and wild-looking Chinese in padded cotton clothes—with long sleeves coming down over their hands and huge long-haired fur caps with flapping earpieces—chickens, and piles of baggage tied up in squares of cotton, I, as the only foreigner, excited considerable curiosity. They gave me a place near the reeking stove, then crowded around to stare, finger my boots, try the laces, and demand where my husband was. I was glad the secretary was with me.

At one station, a group of schoolboys got in and surrounded me to get a look at the pictures in the magazine I was trying to read. I obliged by turning the pages. They looked at all the pictures and asked the English name of everything. Their bright faces were none too clean and all needed handkerchiefs, but nobody had any. In the winter, all Korean children seemed to have runny noses. My traveling companion told the boys to wipe their noses. When they paid no attention, he searched his pockets and finding a bit of old newspaper went the rounds with it. Though cleanliness is said to be next to godliness, I'd never seen a church worker make such a practical demonstration in a public conveyance.

On the south bank of the Tumen, white-robed Koreans carried enormous jiggy loads on their backs or drove bull carts loaded with straw bags of soybeans. On the north bank, blue-clad Chinese trotted along with their heavy baskets swinging from shoulder poles or drove pack ponies, donkeys, or mules.

After satisfying the police at Sambong, we were on our way to an inn when we met Miss Jessie Whitelaw who had come from Yongjung to meet me. With her was a young man by the name of Lee Choon-Chul who had the English name of

Alexander. As he spoke Chinese and Japanese as well as his native Korean, he was a most useful traveling companion.

We spent the night at a Korean home where the Christians met for worship since there was no church. In addition to the food we had, the hostess brought hot water and boiled rice and eggs. Before we could begin to eat, visitors began to arrive. But, as it is bad form in Korea to watch people eat, they faded away till we could have our meal.

After supper, the Christians gathered. The men sat in the kitchen. The women—half of them with babies on their backs—sat with us in the other room. Each room was the standard size: eight-feet square. The secretary from Hoiryung, standing in the doorway between, conducted a service.

Afterward, it appeared Miss Whitelaw had said a doctor would be there that evening and so the people expected an instant clinic. Unfortunately the unsuspecting doctor had little with her that was of much service. However, I looked at all the sore throats, ears, eyes, abscesses and various other infirmities, gave advice through Miss Whitelaw and Alexander, and promised to send necessary remedies from Yongjung.

When at last all had departed, we got out our blankets and made our sleeping places on the floor. Since the outdoor temperature was several degrees below zero and the paper doors and windows seem to admit as much cold as they kept out, we filled a hot-water bottle and lighted two Japanese heaters—small, flat tin cans with tightly fitting covers. A cigar-shaped stick of charcoal, ignited and inserted in the can, burned slowly for several hours and gave considerable heat. These heaters could also be carried in a pocket or under the outer clothing in cold weather.

Another patient arrived before breakfast to be duly prescribed for before we started for Yongjung. It was a twenty-three mile drive and the temperature was eight degrees below zero. Upon arrival at the border we walked to the river and, after showing passports, satisfying the police as to our ages and business, and going through all the red tape dear to the hearts of Japanese officials, we finally passed customs. Though we were entering China and had Chinese visas on our passports, the immigration and customs officials were Japanese. China naturally didn't like this, but such was the state of affairs at that time. As part of the indemnity, the Chinese had to pay for the Boxer Uprising, when many foreigners were killed. Thus Western nations collected the customs for a number of years. I believe, however, that the Japanese were not acting under this reparation agreement, but were there because the Chinese just couldn't stop them.

Crossing the frozen river, we found the carts Alexander had arranged for and made ourselves as comfortable as we could in our blankets. Miss Whitelaw and I were in a Russian cart and Alexander on a flat one with the baggage, blankets, and a hot-water bottle. In that temperature, the wind felt like razors, but our driver drove all day with bare hands.

We started. We stopped for some reason unknown to us. We started again, and again stopped. Soon we had obvious reason to stop: with a steep cliff on one side and the river many feet below on the other, the road was too narrow to pass another team that was approaching at a leisurely pace. After it passed we entered the narrow part of the road again, only to back out once more for other vehicles. Then our driver discovered the broken rim and tire on one of the wheels, which had been patched with a bit of spoke and a piece of straw rope. We waited while repairs were carried out. These soon proved ineffectual and before we reached the next village we were glad to get down and walk rather than be spilled out on the frozen road. I decided the best way to ride in a Russian cart was to walk beside it.

At the village we went into the Chinese customs house to get warm. Here the head man was a Korean who spoke English. When he found I was a doctor, we had another clinic.

When the wheel was well roped, away we went once more.

A high two-wheeled Russian cart, if in good condition, was

the only vehicle in that part of the world with springs and thus a luxurious conveyance. One got aboard by climbing up the spokes of the big wheel and falling into blankets and heaters with as much grace and dignity as possible under the circumstances.

Our steed was a "big horse" as opposed to a Manchurian pony, though he wasn't much larger.

We met a succession of Russian carts, Chinese carts, Korean bull carts, Pekin carts with high canvas covers, pack ponies and donkeys, and Japanese and Chinese soldiers on horseback. Chinese carts were four-wheeled vehicles drawn usually by four Manchurian ponies—sometimes by three ponies with a cow or donkey between the shafts and the others running abreast in front. The ponies were so small and shaggy they looked like a cross between real ponies and sheep. Their tempers were uncertain, and like some humans, they were not to be trusted too far.

Korean carts drawn by large bulls traveled between market towns in groups of a dozen or more laden with straw bags of soybeans, a chief export of Manchuria. No animal ever got off the road till the very last minute, so collisions were avoided (when they were) by an excitingly narrow margin. Korean carts, with hubs projecting a foot beyond the sides, were so heavy and cumbrous that they never sustained damage and hence no care whatever was taken to avoid another vehicle.

Once or twice, while our driver was off on an excursion of his own, the horse went on unsupervised till he met a bull cart. Neither gave way, and there was an impasse until our driver returned and dragged his animal off the road. Drivers led instead of driving from behind, which probably accounted for our comparatively rapid progress, for the beasts had to go as fast as the shouting drivers walked.

To keep warm we frequently got down and walked till the savage barking of dogs warned us we were approaching a village. Since Manchurian canines were watchdogs with a special aversion to foreigners, we would climb the spokes again and collapse into the blankets.

Finally, we stopped at a Chinese inn to get warm and eat our lunch. The door stood invitingly open all the time, admitting fresh air, while the open fire and cooking food added unknown smells and considerable smoke to the atmosphere. Koreans, Chinese, and Japanese in the next room were clamorously feasting. Noisy eating and belching indicated enjoyment and was expected of guests.

The paper windows in our room admitted little light. When our eyes adjusted to the dimness, we saw a raised platform at one side of the room serving as both seat and bed. Chinese couldn't sit on their mud floors as Koreans did on their clean, heated ones, and so they used chairs or benches.

Getting as close as possible to the smoky bit of fire in the tin pail, we tried to warm up.

The kindly landlord picked up the cups left on the table by previous guests, scraped out the tea leaves with a dirty forefinger, flung them on the floor, and poured out more tea from the kettle boiling on the fire. Setting the cups before us, he invited us to drink. I looked at my fellow travelers. Alexander was enjoying his and Miss Whitelaw sipping hers. I let mine get cold and didn't drink it. It takes time to get used to some things. We ate the sandwiches Miss Whitelaw had brought from Yongjung as soon as they thawed out, while several spectators who had come in to watch us eat satisfied their curiosity. The Chinese apparently did not have the custom of leaving people alone to eat, and considered eating with fingers instead of chopsticks unpleasant.

After the mountains of Korea, we found the rolling plains of Manchuria bleak and bare. Large fields were quite unlike the tiny patchwork-quilt paddies south of the Tumen. There was scarcely a tree in sight and the wind swept continuously over the bare, frozen, and deeply cracked soil.

"There," said Miss Whitelaw toward evening, "see that one lone tree over there on that distant hilltop? That's just opposite the town. We're nearly home."

Everyone was present at the station dinner to welcome me: Archie and Mrs. Barker, E. J. O. and Mrs. Fraser, the

Martins, and all the children, Emma Palethorpe, Jessie Whitelaw, and Mary Thomas, a visitor from Sungjin.

It was wonderful to join in the fellowship and be at home somewhere, for at least another year.

-4-

Next morning, Dr. Martin still weak and lame took me over to the hospital. A versatile young man from Newfoundland, he had planned and built the hospital himself. It was better planned, better built, and better equipped than the older mission hospitals I had seen. There wasn't a plumber or electrician in that part of Manchuria, so the doctor had installed plumbing and electric wiring himself. His small generator produced the first electric power in the province. It lighted the hospital, ran the pump to supply the hospital with water, and was to run the portable x-ray machine he expected to bring back with him after his furlough.

Stanley Martin was a man of middle height, thin and pale from his recent illness. He walked with a limp then, though it didn't seem to slow him down any and, later, disappeared. The blue eyes under his shaggy brows missed nothing. And he was rugged. His capable hands could do almost anything. Besides being a good mechanic, he was a qualified wireless operator, amateur astronomer, excellent physician, and competent surgeon. He had a heart full of sympathy for the poor and the suffering.

Six years earlier, he had started and carried on a clinic and performed operations in two rooms of the mission women's house until the hospital was built. His Korean and Chinese excited my admiration and despair.

He had a fine telescope for which he must have sacrificed many things. His enthusiasm for astronomy induced him to drag others of us out into the bitterly cold nights to see the mountains on the moon and its craters, which he said were three hundred miles across.

The only qualified doctor in the district, he had been seeing *twenty-two thousand* patients a year, in addition to administrative work, training staff, and performing surgery. A strenuous undertaking, to say the least. His chief assistant, Deacon Lim, had never seen a medical school. But, trained by Dr. Martin, he could and did diagnose and successfully treat many common medical conditions and perform the simpler operations.

No formal qualifications were necessary for the practice of medicine in Manchuria. Seoul's Severance Medical College was now graduating a few young doctors, but the demand for their services was so great that there were plenty of good positions available in Korea and none wanted to go to Manchuria. Dr. Martin examined the more difficult cases himself and did the major surgery.

Such were the conditions in the early days of mission hospitals. I often wish that these pioneers who struggled with so many difficulties and handicaps could see the fine medical institutions that developed from their unpretentious beginnings.

Making rounds together that first morning, the doctor said, "Koreans prefer their own hot floors to our cold beds when they are sick. That's why several are empty now but the outpatients keep us just as busy throughout the winter as in summer. About half our patients are Chinese."

Approaching a bed where a pigtailed Manchurian was having drops put in his eyes, Dr. Martin turned to me.

"You may as well get your hand in now," he said. "This chap's to have an operation today. You do it."

He introduced me to the patient. "*Nieu daifu*"—woman doctor—he said in Mandarin, the local Chinese dialect.

So I performed my first operation in Yongjung. All went well, fortunately, for otherwise the Chinese would have little confidence in the *nieu daifu.*

I wondered why so many Koreans lived in Manchuria in such unsettled times. The explanation was simple: after 1910 when Japan annexed Korea, they expropriated much of the land in the south where the climate was less severe than farther north. People thus forced off their land moved to Manchuria and Siberia where the population was scanty and land available. Their children, brought up in Siberia under communism, are the communist leaders of North Korea today.

In the earlier stages of their planned conquest of China, the Japanese had also come to Manchuria. They built and controlled the South Manchurian Railway and posted garrisons along the route for its protection. Claiming that all Koreans everywhere were their citizens, they established a consulate in Yongjung under pretext of protecting them. Contrary to their agreement with China, they also stationed a garrison in the city. It was a time of lawlessness and banditry over which the local warlord seemed to have little control. The Chinese one day erected two watchtowers on a hill not far behind our mission houses. They were about twenty feet high but, though the walls were thick, they were of mud and could afford little protection to the sentries. For their own protection the Japanese built a high brick wall around all their property in Yongjung, even closing off some of the main streets. The Japanese had their own school and medical service, which further isolated them, and seldom came to the mission hospital.

The third day after my arrival in Yongjung, Christmas festivities began. It was Saturday, Christmas Eve, and after all the patients were attended to, Dr. Martin gave a dinner for the staff. It was a bitterly cold day with the usual high wind. The only places in the hospital that were comfortably warm were the operating room and Miss Whitelaw's office. Since men and women didn't eat together in Korea, we had to use two rooms.

The men took out the operating table and brought in plain tables, spread with white paper for tablecloths, and ate in the operating room. We made our preparations on the nursing superintendent's desk. A downtown restaurant supplied both Korean and Chinese dishes.

First came a large bowl of chopped meat and vegetables, then a doughy sort of dumpling full of a peppery mixture in a thin broth. Nurses, cooks, laundrywomen, and cleaners, all sat down together with the superintendent of nurses and the newly arrived doctor and set to with brass chopsticks and spoons.

With less than half of what was in my bowl eaten, I began to feel stuffed but there was more to come: cakes, cookies, candies, and a whole box of frozen Mandarin oranges. When all had feasted to capacity the guests gathered up what was left and took it home.

Before fully recovering from this banquet, I went that evening to the missionary station's dinner at Dr. Martin's. For this family occasion, all who were far from home had been invited; among them, Mr. Grierson, a lonely and somewhat recluse Englishman, Mr. Hansen, a Scandinavian, and Mrs. Nadarov, a Russian woman who lived at Kookjaka, about fifteen miles away. After an excellent dinner of pheasant, we played games, heard music, and sang carols.

Christmas day began at four in the morning with carols sung under our windows and outside all the Christian homes in the town by the boys and girls of the mission schools. They came in separate groups, a proper distance apart, and sang in the below zero cold till their throats were hardly fit to take part in the regular Sunday morning service which was a special Christmas celebration. Everybody went. When the church was so crowded that not another person could squeeze through the door, some opened the windows and slipped in.

For many this Sunday was their first Christmas. Some came out of curiosity, others to hear their children sing, the boys on one side of the church, the girls on the other, singing alternately. It was an opportunity to tell what Christmas was all about and the church made the most of it. Santa Claus didn't figure in it. The Christ Child did.

After the Korean Christmas service, Dr. and Mrs. Martin and I were invited to the Chinese church. Here women sat at the back and men in front, on benches that were high, narrow, backless, and most uncomfortable. People kept coming in and going out leaving the doors wide open. Children sang, but this time I failed to recognize the tune. However, the people of this small congregation were doing well. There was no mission station anywhere near and they had no outside help. Our mission worked with Koreans and none of us spoke Chinese except the doctor.

After the service, a number of people gathered at the pastor's house. The women remained in an outer room while the Martins and I, as guests, were led to an inner room with the men.

As usual, the Chinese wore their heavily padded clothes indoors, not having much heat in their houses. Unlike Koreans, they wore their shoes inside and I was glad not to have to remove mine for, as I had discovered, there was nothing colder than shoes that have been refrigerating on the doorstep in zero weather.

Cracks between boards in the floor provided plenty of ventilation so the tiny stove, containing a handful of coals, did little to make its presence known except by the smoke it emitted. The sections of its long, thin stovepipe, I noticed, were held together by bands of paper pasted around the joints, while the end of the pipe stuck out through the paper window. Yet there was absolutely no danger of the window catching fire, for no heat ever reached that far. We sat in our winter coats with our boots on and shivered.

The pastor and his son beamed at us. The colonel in command of Chinese troops in the district was a Christian, as was another guest, an educated Chinese who spoke English well. The wives of these people were very gracious although the language problem restricted conversation.

Most of the older women—but not many of the younger ones—had bound feet. That cruel custom was slowly being overcome but still continued in interior China until the communists put an end to it.

The women of course ate by themselves but, knowing the strange ways of Western people, they had set places for Mrs. Martin and me with the men.

As was the custom, we visited first while the food was prepared, since we knew that Chinese etiquette required a polite exit after eating. Thus, we struggled with conversation for a long time before tea, cakes, cookies, and candy appeared.

While enjoying these snacks, I wondered if this was all that would be served or if we should reserve space for what might come after. Dr. Martin advised an attitude of expectancy, so I refrained from satisfying my appetite though it was past three in the afternoon. The host had the teapot in his hand the whole time, and as soon as there was room for another spoonful in anybody's cup, he poured it in. When the tea in the pot began to cool, he spilled the contents on the floor and sent a servant for more.

When we were all full of tea, we walked around the room, partly to keep warm and partly to shake down the tea to make room for what we now believed was the feast to come.

After another half hour, the women brought in bowls of food and set them on the table. Each was given an individual rice bowl and helped himself as he fancied from the others. With their chopsticks, the host and his friends helped us to specially delectable bits. I hoped no one had tuberculosis. Several kinds of meat and vegetables were prepared in various ways, all in small pieces easily handled with chopsticks. When anyone felt replete, he got up, walked about the room, spit on the floor, and returned to begin again. I counted twenty-one different dishes on the table at once.

Dinner lasted for two hours. We had to tear ourselves away, saying thanks and farewell with much bowing to each person at the top of the stairs, again at the bottom, and once more out at the street. We hastened to get to the Christmas service in our own language at the Martin house and all went again to Korean church that night.

-5-

When Ahn Sunsaing arrived, we settled down to morning study. In the afternoons, we saw patients together in the hospital. He explained to me in my limited Korean vocabulary what the patient had said. I then explained as best I could what I wanted to say to him. Ahn, in turn, relayed this to the sick one and his friends. It was a slow and sometimes rather painful process and I frequently wondered whether the meaning intended was actually conveyed in either case. With Chinese patients translation was even more complicated and Alexander was usually called to interpret.

Russian patients were a different problem as none of our staff spoke their language and they knew no other tongue. These unfortunate people were among the first great group of refugees, having fled for their lives from their native land.

Following the Russian revolution in 1917, the Bolsheviks fought their way eastward, reaching the Pacific coast in 1921, the year I arrived in Asia. White Russians loyal to the czar fled, many in ill-equipped and badly supplied old ships of the Russian Pacific fleet. They appealed to several countries for refuge, including Canada and the United States, but were refused everywhere. Although they were fleeing from the Soviets, other nations feared there might be communists among them.

When food and fuel ran out, they could neither go farther nor remain on board to starve. Finally, they were allowed on shore in various parts of east Asia. Hundreds landed at the Korean port of Wonsan where some of the battles had been fought during the Russo-Japanese War years earlier. Here they spent weeks—ill-clothed and half starved—in barbed-wire enclosures guarded by Japanese soldiers.

Though foreigners in Korea did what they could to help, it was beyond the power of a few hundred to provide for these thousands of destitute people. When Japanese authorities tired of feeding them and didn't know what else to do, they opened the gates of the encampments and told them to fend for themselves.

Similar experiences faced the Russian expatriates in other places. Many eventually found their way to Hong Kong and Shanghai where they made places for themselves in the community. A few, less fortunate or less resourceful, became rickshaw pullers, beggars, or prostitutes. White men pulling rickshaws, begging and sleeping in the streets, was something new in the Orient.

"Ah yah!" observed the Oriental nodding his head, "Maybe the white man is not so superior after all."

Not surprisingly, our Russian patients were malnourished as well as sick. They didn't adjust to the Korean food served in the hospital, and couldn't even tell us what they would like. They were lonely and anxious over their own fate and that of loved ones left behind in Siberia.

One big man, a professional pianist who knew some English, sometimes came as interpreter for his fellow countrymen. Once he accompanied an opera singer ill with pneumonia. She brought her small dog. They explained it couldn't be left behind as it was paralyzed and had to wear diapers.

Our nurses felt they had enough to do looking after sick people and weren't at all pleased at being expected to nurse a dog. Besides, who was going to wash the diapers? I didn't blame them. Neither did Miss Whitelaw. However, patient and dog were both cared for and I didn't ask questions about who was doing what. The singer recovered, the dog didn't.

His mistress gave a concert, dressed in various articles of clothing contributed by the mission women, to express her gratitude.

The nurses didn't like to nurse Russian patients and I once had to reprimand them for not being kinder to one.

"We can't stand the smell of them," they protested.

"Smell!" I exclaimed. "They won't smell if you keep them clean."

"All the Russians smell awful. We hate to go near them. They all smell like weasles."

"Like weasles, do they? If foreigners smell, we must smell too. What do Dr. Martin and I smell like?" I demanded to know.

This was embarrassing, but they finally admitted we smelled like cows. "Don't you drink milk and eat butter and cheese?" they pointed out. "Why wouldn't you smell like cows?"

While struggling with the Korean language and seeing the sick, I also learned something of political conditions. Dr. Martin told me of his experiences during the Japanese punitive expedition following the Korean Independence Movement of 1919. Koreans had heard of Wilson's Fourteen Points during peace discussions in Europe and they thought if only they could let the world know they wanted to be independent again and free from Japan—which had annexed Korea in 1910—the world might do something about it. They planned that on a certain date all over the country they would gather in central places and shout for independence. Unarmed and pledged not to use force no matter what the provocation, they gathered together and shouted *Mansei,* "Long live Korea," or literally "Korea for ten thousand years."

It was amazing that such nationwide arrangements could be made and carried out without the police hearing any whisper of what was afoot. Taken entirely by surprise, the Japanese went into a panic. Police and gendarmes rushed into the crowds with swords and guns. They wounded many, shot some, and arrested and tortured thousands, many of whom were merely bystanders. A few days later the same kind of protests occurred in Manchuria with the same results.

Dr. Martin cared for the injured and hid people sought by the police in his house and at the hospital. He treated the injured and buried those who died from their wounds. He showed me his photographs: long lines of dead laid out in the basement of his hospital. Most of them had had nothing to do with the so-called seditious movement except to shout *Mansei,* which of course every Korean did.

A legal loophole had saved many, Stanley Martin explained. Part of the price imposed on China for the killing of foreigners in the Boxer Rebellion had been "extraterritoriality." This meant that groups of foreigners living in China were not subject to the Chinese courts but were, for all practical purposes, living in a bit of their native land and subject to their own judicial systems. It was an obvious thorn in the flesh of China but at that time a boon to the Koreans. The tiny mission compound was legally entitled to fly the British flag and it did so during the panic. Under it, Dr. Martin was able to shelter Koreans fleeing from the police who could not legally pursue them. Not long after this, extraterritoriality was relinquished. However, Dr. Martin's daring help was one reason he was so loved and respected.

Life at the mission quickly became a comforting routine: Ahn Sunsaing's study hours in the mornings and patients in the afternoons. I discovered I was able to understand and speak a little Korean. My teacher would test my comprehension by telling me stories and then have me repeat them back to him. A favorite concerned his uncle, a tiger hunter who had shot four tigers in the hills not far from Hamheung four years ago. Ahn said the meat tasted much like beef. Indeed, many people liked dog and some ate cat meat. I began to wonder what kinds of meat were in the various dishes I enjoyed at Christmas time. Perhaps it was just as well not to know.

As a change from sitting at a desk, we often went for walks. As in Hamheung and Hoiryung, the city cemetery was near the mission compound and we invariably strolled past. This one had sections for Chinese, Koreans, and Japanese.

Chinese buried their dead in huge coffins made of planks so heavy that it took two horses to move them. They were often chosen by their future occupant who would keep the coffin at home for years. When the time came, the coffin was hauled to the graveyard and left above ground awaiting an auspicious day for burial. When we walked by, there were always about a dozen coffins lying about. Burial consisted of a few shovelfuls of earth thrown over the coffin usually leaving the ends exposed. The many hungry dogs that prowled the hills made the need for heavy coffins obvious.

Koreans, on the other hand, heaped great mounds of earth on graves and the Japanese buried their dead close together in a small plot and erected wooden staves with the name of the departed over them.

In spite of these various measures, we sometimes saw gnawed bones lying about.

Early in February came the Chinese New Year, and a request from the governor of the province for Dr. Martin and the *nieu daifu* to come to Kookjaga, the provincial capital and prescribe for his sick daughter. Mrs. Nadarov also lived there and had invited us, so we combined the two visits. It took most of the day to get there in a Russian cart over the rough frozen road.

We found the girl ill with tuberculosis. We gave instructions about rest, food, and fresh air, and left some medicine. The governor presented us each with a beautiful cloisonné vase.

The Nadarovs, we found, lived in a typical Chinese house of the better class—a long low one-story building with the barn attached at one end. There was no corridor. One room opened into the next, each so packed with furniture and various inventions of Mr. Nadarov that the space between formed a sort of passageway.

Next to the barn was the pantry, beyond it the kitchen, then the dining room, and finally the living room where the precious barometer hung on the wall. Farther on were the bedrooms.

Mr. Nadarov had been a petty consul in this remote region till the revolution in Russia, when he suddenly found himself an enemy of the state, cut off from family and friends and without income. They had to stay where they were and never received any word from or about their friends and relatives, whom they feared had been liquidated (a fate they feared for themselves, even in their isolation).

They had to do something to support themselves. Mrs. Nadarov was an educated woman who spoke several languages, but no one in Kookjaga wanted to learn Russian, English, French, or German—all of which she could have taught. Mr. Nadarov was a scientist who wrote learned articles for scientific journals. He specialized in predicting storms and natural disasters all over the world and showed us his scrapbook made up of reports of storms, earthquakes, and tornados in various parts of the globe that he claimed to have accurately foretold. He studied the skies and believed sunspots told him much. Thus, he refused to leave his house as that might cause him to miss some of his weather observations. He and his wife met only at breakfast and supper, since he stayed up all night to take notes on the weather and she did so by day.

He was also an inventor. The first thing one wanted to do in their house was to find out what the various odd-looking devices were and how to work them. If you wanted a shower bath, there was a button to push, but it was important to know exactly which one. All his gadgets were handmade of wood. Unlike those of the population at large, the Nadarov's sanitary conveniences were indoors. On pulling a string, the toilet bowl flushed. By lighting a bundle of paper placed conveniently nearby, other waste matter was disposed of by burning. On touching a button, towels appeared as if by magic. By touching another, the soap retreated into its receptacle. It was a fascinating house.

After supper, we exercised the Nadarovs' calf and ourselves. As it was too cold to put the creature out, we all stood in the doorway of the living room, with the door open between barn and pantry. In came the calf, racing through the pantry, kitchen, and dining room as fast as its little hooves could carry it. First we heard its hooves clatter on the wooden floor, then as it approached we saw the bright gleam of its two eyes. Then the whole calf came in sight and made a dash for the living room door. Since the barometer was in that room and might be damaged by the prancings of the animal, we in the doorway seized the calf around the neck and turned it about. It galloped happily to the end of the course, then turned and raced back to us. This continued till the novelty wore off for all concerned.

Mrs. Nadarov opened the kitchen window and scraped the dishes out into the backyard for the geese and then we had to see the cows in the barn. One had lost her calf and refused to be milked. Ingeniously, Mr. Nadarov had skinned the unfortunate calf, rolled up the skin, and simply took it to the unhappy mother at milking time. The cow sniffed the skin and as long as it was near there was no further difficulty milking her.

The Nadarovs tried to eke out a living by selling milk, but the Orientals, who had never drunk any, didn't like it. About the only ones who would drink it were tuberculous patients who had heard that milk was good for their affliction. They took it like medicine.

Dr. Martin, in spite of his lame leg, undertook to introduce me to the excitements of the Chinese New Year. We joined the revelers in the streets where for one night bandits and soldiers mingled with the populace in celebration. The crowds sang, shouted, joked, set off firecrackers, dragged paper dragons through the streets, and burned paper money for good luck. No one was afraid. Ragged Chinese soldiers in worn and faded cotton uniforms brushed shoulders with schoolboys, farmers, white-clad Koreans, and Japanese soldiers: a motley crowd intent on making the most of the one big holiday of the year.

Not long after this came the sad news of the death in Hamheung of Dr. Kate MacMillan. An epidemic of typhus fever had spread to the girls in the mission girls' school dormitory. Dr. MacMillan had cared for the sick students day and night. When she herself developed the disease, she had no strength left with which to resist it. She succumbed and was buried in the little foreign cemetery on Dragon Hill beside the mission children and wives who had died far from their native land, but not beyond the love and care of their heavenly Father. Koreans came from near and far to show their love and respect at her funeral.

Dr. Martin was depressed at the news. "You and I will go out like that some day too," he said, but in that he was mistaken.

-6-

Medical practice in Yongjung proved to be very different from that in Canada. Infectious diseases were more or less controlled in the West, but in Korea some diseases I'd never encountered were common: typhoid, typhus, diphtheria, leprosy, malaria, sprue, and many parasitic conditions. Not long before, cholera and plague had invaded Manchuria and were always on my mind although I never saw a case of either. While I was in Yongjung, I saw my first case of epidemic encephalitis, an infectious inflammation of the brain then called sleeping sickness. The very next mail brought a medical journal describing the disease that had appeared at about the same time on the other side of the world.

Tuberculosis of all types and in all regions of the body was the greatest public health problem. Complications often due to neglect, ignorance, or incorrect treatment were both common and more severe than I had ever seen.

Another condition new to me were the tiny deformed feet of Chinese women. One woman from Peking showed me her feet. Chinese were said to call them golden lilies. To me they were a horrible crippling deformity. The toes were bent backward under the sole, the heels pulled forward till the foot of a mature woman was only four inches long. To create this, parents would tightly bind the feet of small girls with bandages. These were gradually tightened in spite of the pain that lasted for weeks or months. Sometimes it caused gangrene. These bandages were kept in place throughout the female's life. It was amazing that anyone could see beauty in such a deformity or that any parent could inflict such suffering on a small child. However, upper-class Chinese feared they would not find suitable husbands for their daughters if they were allowed to have big feet, like servants.

Another explanation was that foot binding made it difficult for wives to run away from cruel husbands or tyrannical mothers-in-law. Though there was beginning to be a sentiment against the practice in China, most of the Chinese women I saw in Yongjung had bound feet and hobbled through life with short, unstable steps.

Chinese who became Christian sometimes tried to unbind their daughters' feet, but that too was a slow and painful process and such feet never became normal. Fortunately for them, the big sturdy Manchurian women had no such cruel custom. They needed strong feet to do the heavy work required of them.

I often saw the serious complications that often followed treatment by people without scientific training. These practitioners often punctured the painful area, or some other part of the body allegedly related to it, with needles. This popular treatment, known as the *chim,* could be carried out in about three hundred locations on the human body. The public had great confidence in it and generally resorted to it before they sought any other form of treatment. These so-called doctors were trained by an apprenticeship to practitioners of the old school whose textbooks were written hundreds of years before.

They used needles with sharp triangular points for puncturing muscles and joints and blunt-pointed ones for boring into the abdomen. Needles might be wiped off on a dirty sleeve and inserted cold, or else heated and used red hot in which case they were at least sterile. Cold needles often introduced infection. The *chim* was used for various conditions as it was generally believed to relieve pain no matter what the cause.

Another treatment favored by patient and practitioner alike was known as the *doom,* an ironically apropriate name. In *doom* treatment, the healer placed little piles of powdered leaves of certain plants on the skin over the affected area and then ignited them. He usually did this many times on the same spot and might treat several such spots at once. The burned tissue sloughed away leaving a deep ulcer through the whole thickness of the skin or even deeper. I asked one woman, whose loss of tissue from the *doom* treatment had penetrated the muscular layer, how many times she had had the *doom* in that spot. One hundred times, she told me. I believed her.

Both *chim* and *doom* treatments often caused serious complications for the surgeon. When a tumor that had been needled several times came to be operated on, adhesions due to the needling made the surgery unnecessarily difficult and increased the risk. If the patient required surgery where there were several dirty, infected *doom* ulcers over the operative area, there was obviously great danger of infection from the sores entering the wound. The results were often disastrous. If possible, I waited till the ulcers healed. In emergencies I sometimes wondered if it wouldn't be better to let the patient die of his ruptured appendix and its complications or his internal hemorrhage, rather than of postoperative infection from his ulcers.

In such cases, I explained to the anxious relatives the problem due to the neglected disease and the infected ulcers, and asked them to decide whether they wished to take the risk of operation under such conditions. I always used such situations to teach people the importance of coming to the hospital before complications occurred and the danger of first having *chim* or *doom* treatment. If they wished to accept the risk and take the responsibility for the result, I would operate and do my best to save the patient. Usually they decided to have the operation.

If there were only a few dirty ulcers along the line of incision, I excised them and hoped for a clean field through which to operate. If there were many, I excised those in the line of incision, cleansed the others as well as I could, and sealed them with collodion gauze in the hope that it would remain in place till healing took place. It didn't always. But, in spite of such hazards, so many patients did well that I was convinced Oriental patients had developed special immunity to many bacterial flora and fauna prevalent in their environment.

The most frequent operation—even then a thing of the past in Western lands—was the removal of suppurating tuberculous lymph nodes from the neck. No drug then available improved that condition, while overcrowding, the common habit of spitting everywhere, and general unsanitary conditions promoted its spread. It was important to remove such nodes before they ruptured due to secondary infection from other bacteria took place. Such mixed infections took months to heal if they ever did and always left unsightly scars. *Chim* or *doom* treatment, by introducing such secondary infection, made eventual surgery difficult and the result less than perfect.

Most such patients already had open running sores on both sides of the neck. As the inflamed nodes were invariably adherent to large nerves and blood vessels, the operation was difficult and long.

When women, who didn't like going to a male doctor, heard there was a medical woman at St. Andrew's Hospital, they began coming to see me in such numbers that it curtailed my time for language study; and patients unable to come to the hospital begged for house calls. This is a simple matter where doctors have cars and paved roads. Since I had to walk everywhere, it took more time. Listening to lengthy and often irrelevant accounts of the sick person's complaints was also time-consuming and five house calls were about as many as I could make in an afternoon.

The first woman I saw in her home had suffered from tuberculosis of the hip for three years and the disease had spread through her entire body. I'd never seen anyone so thin and twisted. She suffered constant pain and her condition was now quite hopeless. She was lying on the floor entirely helpless, a few rags on top of her and not much beneath. The outside temperature was twenty degrees below zero and seemed to be little more inside. My teeth were chattering from the cold. To keep from freezing, her small son—whose only clothing was a short jacket—lay under his mother's ragged bedding. There was no one but her husband to do anything for her and the two little ones. Though the husband worked hard, most of his wages went to buy condensed milk for his wife who could take nothing else, and it was very expensive in Yongjung.

Our nurses made clothes for the family and bathed and dressed mother and children, whose gratitude was pathetic to see. The poor woman's sufferings soon came to an end, for she died a few days later.

On another occasion, I went to a Chinese home to see a man ill with tuberculosis. I happened to know that his brother was suffering from syphilis in an infective stage. Kim Sunsaing from the hospital accompanied me as interpreter since he spoke a little Chinese.

At the house, instead of going at once to see the sick man, we were invited to sit down in an outer room where the hospitable master of the house lighted the family pipe and handed it to me. I didn't know what Chinese etiquette decreed in such cases and feared it might be taken as a slight if I refused. Even had I been a smoker, the family pipe in that house would have had no attraction for me. I declined as politely as I could. The man then lighted a cigarette, took a puff to get it going well, and passed it to me. Again, at the risk of giving offense, I had to decline.

He then emptied the used teacups onto the floor, poured fresh hot tea, and gave cups to us. Kim accepted his. Fearing to decline a third time, in spite of unhappy thoughts about the infectious diseases in the household, I forced myself to swallow a few drops. The hardships that friends of overseas missionaries sometimes deplore are often more subtle than they imagine.

One evening Miss Whitelaw and I crossed the river to see some sick Koreans on the other side. In one house a woman with a new baby was lying on the kitchen floor in a room about three feet by six. The other room, six by six feet, was occupied by five people. It was neat and reasonably clean.

As in all Korean houses, the mud floor of the kitchen was about eighteen inches lower than that of the rest of the house. Soup and rice pots were set into the kitchen floor above the fireplace, and flues led under the upper floor. Thus, the one fire cooked the food and warmed the floor of the rest of the house as well as providing the sole source of heat. A hole in the wall at the opposite end of the house, a couple of feet above the ground, permitted the smoke to escape.

Some families added a bit of iron pipe to make a chimney. Others made them of mud and straw matting or a few bits of board. However, these chimneys didn't make much difference to those in the house, but were a boon to passersby as they carried the smoke above eye level. The quantities of dust and smoke in the atmosphere no doubt helped to account for the frequency of eye diseases.

We did what we could for the sick. Sometimes they needed food, sometimes medicine, sometimes instruction and sympathy. The hospital evangelist often went with me on these home visits and followed up, bringing what was needed and giving council and encouragement, as well as preaching the Gospel of the love and mercy of God. The church people often helped out in cases where home care was needed for the children during the illness of the mother, or provided food or clothing. Many people experiencing this kindly concern and help from strangers became interested in their motives for doing it, and often they, too, decided to become Christians.

A sad case was that of a Chinese boy who came to the

hospital with a badly infected compound fracture of the leg. We explained to the father that to save the child's life the gangrenous leg should be amputated. The father wouldn't consent until he had discussed the matter with the relatives, especially the man who had bought the boy. This man, "the other father" they called him, refused his consent and took the lad away to suffer great pain and die of the infection.

By March, I was operating every day, Dr. Martin assisted with the more difficult cases. Together we started a system of improved medical records, beginning with the surgical cases. The records till that time did not provide enough detailed information to be of much scientific value. One of the first operations to be fully written up was that of a woman from whom I removed a cyst containing fifteen gallons of fluid. She looked and felt as though about to burst. A mass that large could not be removed through an ordinary incision; first, I had to aspirate much of the fluid to reduce the size of the tumor. As a result of diligent *chim* treatment, the cyst walls firmly adhered everywhere to the surrounding structures. With the tumor, the patient lost about half her body weight. Greatly relieved to be rid of the weight and pressure on her other organs, she left the hospital rejoicing in her restored health and in the Christian faith she had found in the hospital.

Another woman, who had suffered from tuberculosis of the kidney for three years, was in constant distress and without bladder control. The diseased kidney was so much enlarged that I had great difficulty reaching the vessels supplying blood to the organ in order to tie them off before removing the kidney.

The anesthetist at this operation was the son of the Chinese pastor and spoke no Korean, which added to the problem. If I wanted the patient to have more or less anesthetic during the operation I couldn't make my wishes known. However, I succeeded in removing the offending organ and the patient recovered satisfactorily. Surgery under such conditions was quite a strain and a good result had its corresponding satisfaction.

While Dr. Martin was in Yongjung we consulted on difficult cases and often assisted one another.

A young man, whose chest was covered with *doom* scars, came to us one day with the left side of his chest so full of fluid there was no room for air in the left lung. The fluid had pushed the heart so far to the right that the other lung was badly compressed and he was gasping for breath, turning blue in the face.

I removed much of the fluid through a hollow needle and he was greatly relieved. But I had to repeat the aspiration a few times until the fluid finally disappeared. This common condition was due to tuberculous pleurisy. Without an x-ray apparatus, it was impossible to know just how much the disease had affected the lung. Since there was no drug effective for the disease, there was not much more we could do.

He went home rejoicing; several weeks later he returned accompanied by his father to report he had gained health and strength and all the weight he had lost. They had come a long distance on foot to thank us and bring us a dozen eggs in a dirty cloth. Doctors in the West get bigger fees, but have no more grateful patients.

Totally blind for a year and a half from cataracts, another man came to have his sight restored. When I removed the dressings after the operation on the first eye, the patient shouted in great excitement, "I can see! I can see! Aren't there three people here? And they're moving! I can count fingers."

I was almost as happy as he. He came to us blind, full of superstition and in fear of evil spirits, whom he suspected of having brought his blindness upon him. He left with sight restored, and his fear gone since he now knew that the Great Spirit, God, loved and cared for him and was more powerful than any evil spirit.

One cold winter day a little cavalcade of fourteen men wearing topknots and black horsehair hats with heavy padded white cotton clothing brought a patient from a distant village in the hills. He was lying on a rough stretcher made from saplings covered with straw bags.

"Sal lyo chusio," ("Save him.") they pleaded. "How long will it take to cure him?"

"How long has he been sick?" I asked.

"A long time."

"How long? Two years?"

"Who knows how long? Give him an injection right away. Will he be well in a week?"

"I'm afraid he'll never be well. You should have come sooner."

He was wasted away to skin and bone, exhausted by a racking cough, both hips contracted and motionless, while pus was constantly discharging from both thighs. It was obvious he had not much longer to live.

Even when, as in this case, we could do nothing for the sick —especially when we could do nothing—we tried to teach something in hope of having the next patient brought sooner. I tried to explain about infection and the advantage of bringing the sick to the hospital while they still had strength to recover. The young people and those with some education usually understood and put some of this advice into practice, but the older men neither listened nor understood.

I said the sick man could have been helped if he had come in time, but it was now too late. They didn't listen, but started back to their village with their dying friend saying that it wasn't much of a hospital that couldn't cure a sick man.

The topknots marked these villagers as being from a remote place with little contact with modern ideas. Most Korean Christians in those days cut off their topknots to indicate they were leaving the old way of life and entering a new one. Non-Christians often cut theirs as a sign of modernization or because they saw others who had been to the city were doing so. Gradually, the custom died out until after a few years not many topknots were left except in isolated villages where the aged men clung to the old ways. Some, even after discarding the topknot, still wore the horsehair hat. Without the topknot to keep it in place, you would sometimes see a dignified old gentleman with a long white beard wearing his hat at an amusingly rakish angle.

I was once surprised to see a boy of about twelve years of age wearing these symbols of manhood. He was, I discovered, a married man and thus entitled to wear both topknot and hat.

I'm afraid I stared at a young man waiting for his ailing wife when I saw him remove his hat outside the rear entrance, take down the long hair in his topknot, and wash it in a tin basin. He then dried his hair in the wind and twisted it erect again into the traditional knot on top of his head. Next he applied a tight horsehair band, about four inches wide, around his head. This kept the hair in place so it didn't need any attention again for several months. He topped this with a horsehair cap containing a special compartment to accommodate the topknot, and over that went the hat, kept in place by long strings tied under the chin. Or, if the owner was well-to-do, he might have a string of amber beads or an amber pendant hanging from the ties.

During this time, the Martins were preparing to go on furlough. Lim Chipsa, Dr. Martin's trained assistant, was seeing most of the male patients while I saw the female ones. Miss Whitelaw's nurses did good work and Alexander's capable fingers did many of the dressings in the dispensary. He interpreted for Chinese patients, talked to the Japanese, and spoke English to me. He did a good deal of the laboratory work and was talented in painting on silk and as a singer. His handwriting was as even as print. Alexander wanted to study medicine in Seoul at Severance Medical College, but Dr. Martin arranged for him to help me until he himself should return from furlough the next year.

I was now reasonably fluent in the language and, though many of the village people used a sort of dialect with various colloquialisms, still I understood most of what they said.

On meeting someone I was usually first asked, "How old are you?" This was not rude, but merely showed a polite interest in me. My blond hair was so unnatural looking to them that they thought it must be faded and I must be quite old. They often guessed my age at least twenty years more than it was. On being told I was twenty-eight, one woman remarked in surprise, "And you're nice looking yet," for most native women at that age would already have several children and be worn out from hard work and poverty.

Predictably, the second question would be, "How old is your son?" or, "How many sons have you?" They were amazed to find that at my advanced age I wasn't even married.

"Surely your parents must have died when you were very young," they would say, "that you hadn't anyone to arrange a marriage for you."

They were still more astonished to find that in our country parents let their offspring choose their own life partners and that some choose to remain unmarried.

Women often came and asked to be shown through our house. We welcomed these contacts and always showed them around. The conveniences in the kitchen surprised them: fire in a stove that didn't smoke, and a cupboard for dishes. Such luxury! They were amazed at the beds. Weren't we afraid of falling out? And weren't we cold not sleeping on a nice, hot floor?

A Korean woman speaking to a group at the church told her audience, "Soon after the missionaries came to Yongjung, I was left a widow with four young children to bring up. I had nothing and had to go to work. But I had no training or skill of any kind and I didn't know what to do. A friend advised me to try to get a job at one of the mission houses. I was horrified. I could never go there, I thought. Why, they wore their shoes in the house! How dirty they must be. And I even heard—I could hardly believe it—but I heard that they actually had their toilet *in the house.*"

But after checking the premises she understood and asked for a job.

Likewise some Western ideas of Oriental life proved quite inaccurate too.

Though work went on in the hospital as usual, conditions in the country were not quite as usual.

Bandits frequently raided villages on the plain surrounding Yongjung. Several times at night we saw the flames of burning hamlets where the inhabitants had tried to save some of their crops from the marauders and had their village burned down as punishment.

People were moving into the town for protection and shelter after losing their homes and crops. It was commonly said that most of the bandits were Chinese soldiers in the army of the current local warlord, Chang Tso Lin. When their pay went too long in arrears, or they failed to receive their rations, they went and foraged for themselves—conduct not unknown in other armies. When it suited them, they would be soldiers again. In their ragged cotton uniforms they looked more like bandits than soldiers anyway. Sometimes they didn't even pretend to be bandits, but robbed the poor farmers as soldiers.

All too soon for me came the time for the Martin family to leave on furlough. Koreans, Chinese, and foreigners all gave them a great send-off, and presented them with farewell gifts, including a large red silk banner with the doctor's praises written in black on it in large Korean letters and Chinese characters.

I watched them leave in the carts that would take them to the river and then turned to the hospital that was now my responsibility.

Two of the women missionaries left on furlough soon after. The Barkers, too, left for the Wonsan Beach summer resort for Mrs. Barker was suffering from sprue. This chronic debilitating illness was common among foreigners in the East at that time, and there was no known remedy.

Mr. Scott, having been appointed principal of the mission boys' academy, also left to visit other mission schools and confer with the principals before the schools closed for the holidays. This general exodus left Miss Whitelaw and me alone on the station.

About that time, word came from the church board in Canada of a deficit in church finances that had resulted in a cut in our mission budget, including the hospital grant. The previous month's hospital balance was only four dollars. To have even that much we had had to wring every cent we could from the sick. We felt somewhat shamed, but knew we could not pay the staff or purchase supplies on a deficit. The cut was especially disastrous as the roof, a temporary one, was leaking badly and needed to be replaced.

In July, Miss Whitelaw and I went to Wonsan Beach to the annual obligatory mission meeting and, while there heard that four-hundred bandits had attacked a small town ten miles from Yongjung. They had burned down fifty Chinese, several Korean, and two Japanese homes, the Japanese consulate, post office, and arms magazine from which they took many weapons, including several machine guns and much ammunition. Scores were injured and several killed.

I succeeded in getting a doctor to go to Yongjung for Lim Chipsa, who though an excellent assistant, was not a qualified doctor. When the new doctor arrived in August, Lim gave notice with tears in his eyes. It wasn't easy to be supplanted by a newcomer, but we finally succeeded in persuading Chipsa to stay and we all worked together very harmoniously for some months before I had to go to Seoul on business.

During that trip, I developed pneumonia and was so ill that the Severance doctors insisted I should not return to the heavy responsibilities in the North. Much to my regret I had to spend several weeks in the capital, while the new doctor and Lim Chipsa carried on in St. Andrew's Hospital.

-7-

After the death of Dr. Kate MacMillan, the work of the Cheihei hospital in Hamheung had fallen off. Dr. Pak didn't have the reputation of *Maing Pouine,* and finally the mission closed the institution. As there was a qualified doctor in Yongjung and Dr. Martin was expected soon, the mission transferred me to Hamheung to reopen the facility.

Since recent laws regulated building construction, including width of corridors, number of stairs, and other details, we had to make certain changes before we could call the place a hospital or admit more than ten patients.

Thus, my first task on being appointed to Hamheung as superintendent of Cheihei Hospital (Grace Hospital) was to plan and oversee alterations in the building, a job for which a medical course made no provision. As I could find neither blueprints nor other plans of the building, I had to take measurements and make scale drawings from which to work. While necessary changes were being made in the building, I hoped to make some other improvements as well. As funds were limited, it took much planning to work out the best possibilities. In this task, Reverend Duncan McRae, one of the founders of the mission in 1898 and then living in Hamheung, gave much help and encouragement.

We widened the narrow corridor, placed transoms over the doors to admit more light to the passageway, and put in a ramp instead of the step, over which people used to stumble. We moved partitions to make three small rooms into a larger ward where one nurse could observe eight patients at once. This gave us two "big" wards, one on each floor. Other small rooms could be used as private, semiprivate, or isolation rooms as needed.

Hoping to have electricity before long, we installed wiring. A plumber from Seoul put in plumbing to provide running water and sanitary facilities. He also connected up the hot water radiators properly. Some of the radiators had been connected to the furnace and not to the waste pipe, others to the waste pipe but not to the furnace. Now, for the first time, all the radiators conducted heat.

The furnace heated water for hospital use during the winter. We put in a small heater to provide hot water in the summer and installed washtubs in the basement.

A further improvement was a new operating room on the north side of the building, away from the glare of the summer sun. This was larger than the old one and had a composition floor that was less tiring for the feet than concrete and easier to clean.

We acquired some new furnishings and equipment. The old wooden beds, with fine hiding places for bedbugs were replaced with metal ones—crude and clumsy, but still an improvement. The nursing attendants made new mattress covers and the boys filled them with fresh straw. Old stained and worn sheets became cleaning cloths and were replaced with new ones of unbleached cotton. This soon bleached and wore better, in addition to being cheaper than white. Fresh rice husks filled new pillowcases to make hard, unyielding pillows that patients liked better than soft Western ones.

The former staff had dispersed: some had gotten other jobs and most of the girls had married, while Dr. Pak had set up practice in another town. Only six former employees returned—three girls, a youth named Yum Nu-ka, the former errand boy, and Dr. MacMillan's assistant Kang Do-Ka, matron of the nurses' dormitory. I wasn't disappointed. I thought a new staff could be taught to work under different conditions and with improved standards could learn to change their ways. I hoped to start afresh. Dr. MacMillan, struggling alone, had done nobly. But twenty years later, I thought some advances should be possible.

Severance Hospital had a training school for nurses conducted by Esther Shields, who had welcomed us to Korea. I appealed to them for a graduate nurse and one responded. She didn't look very sturdy but nonetheless set to work with the others getting things ready for opening the hospital. She didn't have much energy and, when she had a lung hemorrhage one morning, she admitted suffering from tuberculosis which she thought was cured. After a few days rest, she left for home.

My faithful language teacher, Ahn Sunsaing, and the capable interpreter Alexander Lee from Yongjung both entered Severance Union Medical College as students that year, 1923. It was gratifying but I missed not having their help at Cheihei.

Because I hadn't passed the third-year language examination, the mission employed another young man to instruct me. Lee Sunsaing was a gentle youth whose pleasant smile revealed as beautiful a set of teeth as I've ever seen, even among Koreans who have remarkably fine teeth. He had bright eyes that became narrow slits when he laughed and, like Ahn Sunsaing, he was an excellent teacher possessed of infinite patience. His obliging disposition made him useful in many ways. He became my secretary, purchasing agent for the hospital, business manager, and when we acquired a new sterilizer he ran that, too. He still bears the scars of his devotion to duty when one day the gasoline stove for heating the apparatus blew up and he carried the flaming equipment outdoors in his bare hands.

As language study and surgery didn't mix, I decided to have Lee Sunsaing give the anesthetic while I operated. The first time I explained as well as I could what to do and what to look out for, since he had never even seen an anesthetic administered. I started the anesthesia myself and when the patient was well under the influence, I turned him over to Lee Sunsaing. Then I scrubbed up and did the operation with one eye on the surgery, the other on the anesthetic. Both were successful, and Lee became the official anesthetist for the hospital and, with the simple apparatus available then, a capable one. During the twenty years he acted in that capacity, he never had a fatality. Considering that many of our patients were poor risks and emergency facilities were of the simplest sort, that is a splendid record. It is not much fun to have to stop in the midst of a serious operation to resuscitate a patient. With Lee Sunsaing at the head of the operating table, that didn't often happen.

With hospital renovations completed, I moved into one of the empty rooms and, with the aid of the nursing staff, laid out the equipment and stocked the supply room, nursing stations, and wards.

When another graduate nurse came from Severance, she and Kang Do-Ka began to teach the new assistants their duties. They started by showing them what a faucet was for and that it had to be turned off again after using, as well as how to make beds, give baths, and take temperatures.

Before preparations were complete and the official opening still a few days off, the first patient arrived with a badly fractured leg late one afternoon after the staff had gone home. He had been cutting wood in the mountains when a tree had fallen on his thigh. The leg was badly crushed, the ends of the broken bone sticking out of a jagged wound.

Explaining that we weren't ready for patients yet, we advised him to go to the government hospital.

"I've come a long way to get to *Maing Pouine's* Hospital," he said, "and now I'm here I'm not going any further." With that his friends carried him in and set down the rude stretcher on which he lay inside the front door.

The hospital was for the sick and injured and here was one of them. From what we knew of the government hospital, we thought the staff there would be likely to do no more for the patient than we could.

I gave him an injection to relieve the pain, cleansed the limb as best I could, painted the skin with antiseptic, and reduced the fracture. There was no x-ray apparatus to check on the position of the broken bone, but it seemed to be satisfactory. Infection would be the great problem. Such open fractures were invariably infected. I put the leg up in extension for the night with makeshift splints and the patient was soon more comfortable than he had been since the accident.

The family, under strict orders not to interfere with the leg, stayed with him. The nurse and Kang Do-Ka had come in to help, and next day Yum Nu-Ka was on duty as well. The Cheihei Hospital, Kate MacMillan's Hospital, was open again.

Of thirty beds, ten were ready for occupancy a week later and three already had patients. The graduate nurse from Severance was in charge during the day but, until we could get and train more hospital attendants, the families looked after the patients at night.

A few days after the opening, a thin, dark, middle-aged woman, with an anxious look on her kindly face and softly curling hair, applied for a job. She was a widow with a young daughter to support and educate and was willing to work even in a hospital. Since she could read and write and agreed to work at night, I engaged her on the spot and she went on duty that evening.

For the next six months, the new night nurse and I spent the hours from seven till midnight together in the hospital. She had everything to learn, but she was eager and soon was able to distinguish between internal medications and external applications, how and when to use antiseptics, and how to handle sterile dressings with sterile forceps. She learned how to fill a hot water bottle and place it outside the blanket to prevent burning a patient. She learned to observe those in her care closely and note any change in their condition. After midnight, if anyone needed me, she called. Being older than the other attendants gave her more authority with the patients and their relatives and the wards were quiet and orderly when the assistant night nurse was on duty. However, her eyesight was so poor she could never read a thermometer and someone in the ward had to do it for her so she could enter it carefully on the chart. She became a faithful and reliable assistant nurse who stayed awake and on the job —a great improvement over home attendants.

During rounds one night, I couldn't find the male attendant on duty on the men's floor and discovered him asleep in one of the beds in the big ward. Awakening him, none too gently I'm afraid, I demanded why he wasn't on the job.

"I visited all the wards on the floor," he said "and gave a drink of water to anyone who wanted it. What more is there to do?" he innocently asked.

He was a conscientious person as it turned out, and even newer to his job than the night nurse on the women's floor. When he understood his work and responsibility, he became a reliable member of the staff.

Just as things seemed to be going nicely, I heard that our one and only graduate nurse from Severance was charging the patients for her services. That would never do, yet if I dismissed her, where could I get another trained nurse? Perhaps if I told her kindly that this wasn't allowed and didn't make her lose face, she might mend her ways and could stay with us.

I called her to my office and asked if what I'd heard was true. She admitted it, saying that at Severance all the nurses were allowed to take money from the patients and she supposed it would be the same here. This, I knew, was not true.

I told her that the hospital paid the staff and that no one was to take money from the patients. With this understanding I told her that if she returned the money this time and in the future didn't take any no one need know of the incident and she could continue working in the hospital.

She said she hadn't wanted to take the money, but the old man in Room 5 had urged her to take it until she was ashamed not to. She had the money in her purse, the exact same five one-yen bills. She hadn't spent it because she was unhappy about having taken it and meant to give it back.

"That's fine," I said. "Go and give it back to him now and everything will be all right."

"I can't do that," she said, "but I'll bring the money to you and you can give it back."

She brought the money and the old man, unable to pay more than a small portion of his hospital bill, was glad to have his five yen returned.

The nurse walked out the front door and never entered the hospital again. For ten days she ate and slept in the nurses' dormitory and spent the days going about from house to house in the city telling people that I was a thief. I'd made her pay five yen of her own money when she had already returned that amount to a patient who insisted she take it. Her conscience was clear, but the foreign doctor at the Chei-hei Hospital was nothing but a thief.

There was no way of knowing how many believed this tale, and it was with considerable relief that I heard she finally left the city ten days later.

Experience is a hard but efficient teacher. Henceforth I made sure there was a witness at every interview. Perhaps, in my position, saving my own face, was as necessary as saving that of the culprit.

When our third trained nurse came, she proved to be a tiny, delicate-looking girl with fine silky black hair, not coarse and straight like so many, but with a slight natural wave. Her features were plain and her face so colorless that she looked almost fragile. Though she walked with an habitual stoop, she was as quick and dainty in her movements as a butterfly. Nurse Woo never once failed me during the years we worked together.

After sterilizing the instruments and making all preparations for an operation, she would scrub with me and act both as scrub nurse and first assistant, and I never had a more capable assistant even after there were other doctors on the staff who assisted at surgery. Nurse Woo always knew what I needed and often put it in my hand before I asked for it. She had a keen sense of humor too and we had many a good laugh together over some absurd incident or ridiculous misunderstanding of language. When we finally parted company, it was to let a new, young missionary nurse have the benefit of Nurse Woo's capable assistance in starting public health in the North.

As dispensary patients increased in number and the wards filled up, Nurse Woo needed help, but graduate nurses were few and girls with any education didn't want to work in a hospital. Widows and deserted wives who might be reduced to working in such a place were almost all illiterate. When a young woman who'd had three years in elementary school agreed to work as a nursing attendant, I engaged her. I thought she would be able at least to read the thermometer and fill out the charts. After three days, she came with her nose in the air and said she thought anyone with her education should have a better job than working in a hospital. That was the end of her.

Nurse Woo, the pharmacist, the women nursing attendants, and the cook lived in a thatched mud house next door to the hospital, with Kang Do-Ka as matron.

On Christmas Eve the pharmacist and I attended a Christmas celebration at a little mud church across the river. It was a joyous occasion and we came home in a happy state of mind remembering whose birthday we were commemorating. I was thinking with gratitude of the many in this land who had come to know and follow Him.

The pharmacist was a big, sturdy, plain-looking girl just out of pharmacy school. She seemed to take little interest in her work and I'd discovered more than one mistake she had made. Though I admonished her several times, her work failed to improve. The mission station, acting as a hospital committee, had to approve all new appointments or dismissals. They agreed that mistakes in dispensing could not be tolerated and that the pharmacist should be given notice, but advised waiting till Christmas was past.

About two o'clock that night Do-Ka awakened me from a sound sleep, crying, "Get up, quick! The pharmacist had a fight with the cook and tore her clothes half off. Now she's dragging her to the police station."

Thrusting my feet into bedroom slippers, I slipped on a dressing gown over my nightdress and set off in the snow in pursuit. What a dreadful thing to happen at a Christian hospital on Christmas Eve of all times!

Outside the gate there wasn't a sign of them. The moonlight glistened on the snow and the frosty air was keen. I hurried on toward the police station, but there wasn't a soul in sight. Had they already gone in? I didn't know, but I could hardly follow any further in my state of undress.

Back in the nurses' home I heard the disgraceful story. The staff had been paid early in order to have money for Christmas. The pharmacist had hidden part of her salary in her room. After returning from church, she counted it and declared some was missing. Someone had stolen her money. When all denied it, she made them cast lots to find the guilty one. The lot fell on the cook, whom the pharmacist immediately accused of the theft. Again the cook denied taking the money or knowing anything about it, whereupon the husky young woman fell upon the older one, struck her repeatedly, and tore her clothes. The others, much distressed, tried to stop the girl from beating the cook, but the pharmacist was furiously angry and they couldn't stop her. When she dragged the unfortunate cook into the street, they sent for me.

By the time I had heard this shameful account, the two returned, disheveled and out of breath.

I reminded them it was Christmas morning, a time of peace and goodwill, and no accusations nor quarreling could be tolerated. A young woman beating up an old one was against all custom. There must be no more trouble during

Christmas and next day an inquiry would be made into the affair.

The carolers were around during the night and early morning as usual, but we hardly heard them. Christmas wasn't a happy day for any of us on the hospital staff.

Next morning, Mr. McRae gave his time and wisdom to help solve the difficulty. The pharmacist repeated her story of missing her money, casting lots, and the lot falling on the cook which convinced her of the latter's guilt.

"What do you know about the pharmacist's money?" Mr. McRae asked the cook.

"I needed it," she replied.

"Why did you take it?"

"I didn't take it."

"What did you do with the money?" he asked.

"I bought clothes for my grandchildren with it."

"Then, why did you say you didn't take it?"

"Does an ignorant old woman like me know what she's saying?"

"Did you take the money?" he demanded sternly.

"No."

"Then what happened to it?"

"I bought candy for my grandchildren with it."

"But you said you didn't take it."

"I didn't."

"Where is it? Go and get it."

"I can't. I spent it while the pharmacist was in church."

"Tell the truth. Where's the missing money?"

"Does an ignorant old woman like me know what she's saying?"

So it went on for a considerable time and in the end the truth never was discovered. I wondered if the cook were an ignorant old woman or a pretty smart one.

To prevent further strife, the dismissal of the pharmacist, already decided upon, now seemed urgent. The money had not been found, nor had the cook cleared herself. Both were in the fight and neither would give assurance she wouldn't fight again if opportunity offered. We gave both notice to leave.

The cook left peaceably with or without the missing money. The pharmacist raised a great row, shouting and storming, accusing me of injustice and declaring I had ruined her life. I had made her lose so much face that she could never get another job and no one would ever marry her. It was all my fault.

Mr. McRae came to my aid. He explained that her dismissal was for unsatisfactory work (she'd several times been admonished). Giving her notice had been postponed until after Christmas so as not to interfere with a happy holiday, but this decision had been made before. Also, the decision was not the superintendent's action, but that of the mission station. The row with the cook proved that the pharmacist wasn't a suitable person to have on the staff.

Her friends took to coming to see me at all hours to protest my unfair behavior and demand that she be reinstated. Her brother daily wrote abusive letters which I ignored. This went on for days.

One night after I'd finished night rounds and was getting ready for bed, Do-Ka came to my door saying the brother had arrived on the late train and was downstairs demanding to see me—at once.

"He's in a furious temper," she said. "Whatever you do, don't go down to talk to him alone tonight. He might hurt you."

"Tell him I'm going to bed, and this is no time for an interview. The patients are asleep and we can't have a disturbance in the hospital at this hour. If he has anything to say to me, let him come during office hours and I'll see him."

When Do-Ka delivered this message, the man rushed upstairs to my door which I had locked. He shouted at me through the door. I told him I would see him at a proper time and place, but not in my bedroom at midnight. There was no such custom as he well knew. After some threats, he went away.

Next morning I saw the woman's brother in my office, with Lee Sunsaing and the hospital evangelist present. He had cooled off a little during the night and was decidedly less belligerent. The men helped to calm him down further. We informed him that the decision would not be changed. We asked how he thought his sister would continue working in the hospital after making such a to-do that half the city knew of her dismissal. Wasn't it best, we asked, for her to go quietly and learn from this experience? The brother left considerably subdued and made no more trouble.

Ten years later, the former pharmacist called me to treat her sister in their village several miles away. The sister had typhoid fever during the usual summer epidemic and was very ill. There had been several deaths in the village from the disease and the family was worried. There was no effective treatment and few people knew of or had faith in preventive innoculations. They had no idea that the disease was spread by unsanitary conditions causing pollution of wells that were often situated close to outdoor toilets.

If they heard of a number of deaths in the same village, the Japanese police, who were the public health officers, considered the sickness must be infectious. They came and burned the bedding and other articles in the room where the patient was—a loss the family felt they couldn't afford. As the police never explained the reason for what they did, they failed to gain the cooperation of the populace, who responded by trying to hide such deaths. The victims were often ordered to be cremated, a method of disposal of the body repugnant to the relatives, or the coffin might be ordered to be lined with zinc which added much to the cost.

I treated the girl, who recovered, and neither the former pharmacist nor I referred to our previous relationship, though I sometimes wondered if she too remembered that unhappy Christmas. Later, both women came to thank me, bringing two strings of eggs as payment.

Things seemed to be going pretty well in the hospital when the registrar resigned. I asked the hospital evangelist if he could suggest a reliable man for the position. He gave me a name and when I asked two or three others their opinion of this man for the job, there was a definite lack of enthusiasm. When we engaged someone else, the evangelist congratulated me on the choice and said that his choice would not have been at all suitable.

"Then," I demanded in astonishment, "why did you recommend him? If you tell me one thing last week and another today, how can I know when to believe you?"

"He asked me to recommend him. How could I refuse?"

So I learned another lesson about life and work in Korea —not to take the advice of one person only who may not be disinterested or may have an ax to grind.

Sickness can strike the doctor as well as others, and did. I had to spend three days in bed with influenza. Fortunately, there was no one in very serious condition in the wards just then, but who would run the clinic? Nurse Woo rose to the occasion. There was no one else to do it. She reported to me that night.

She diagnosed a case of common amoebic dysentery and prescribed the only treatment available. She had treated a small child with fluid in its chest. Having seen me draw off fluid, she did the same, carefully inserting the needle in the same spot. I was appalled when she told me, but the parents were pleased, the child's distress relieved, and the little girl made a good recovery. Others were run-of-the-mill cases and Nurse Woo handled them well.

No sooner was Nurse Woo gone than a gentle knock on the door announced the arrival of Kang Do-Ka.

"Pouine, tae tan ham nika?" ("Are you very sick?") she asked me with concern and began to massage my arms. I protested that she must be tired and needn't do that.

"I always did this for *Maing Pouine,"* she said. "It rested her and helped her to sleep, and when she was dying she wanted nothing and nobody but me. 'Where's my old woman?' she kept asking in her delirium. 'Where's my old woman? I want Do-Ka.' I always did this for her and I'm going to do it now for you."

As her gentle, firm hands soothed my flesh, she told me her story.

"When I was a young woman," she said, "I lived in Wonsan where my family was much respected because they were nobility. My husband was an official and I was known as Kang Pouine (Lady Kang). We had a cook and a maid and I didn't have to do any work, but gave my time to our three little sons and daughter. We were happy till three of the children died of a throat disease that choked them to death within two days of each other. Many children died that way then, for there were no doctors nor hospitals in those days. Everyone thought sickness was caused by evil spirits and they used to hire a *mudang* (sorceress) to drive them away. The spirit causing the disease was so strong, the *mudang* couldn't drive it away and my children died." Do-Ka smiled ruefully. "That's how ignorant we were. I was desolate and cried day and night for my little ones, till a friend whose only son died then too, came to comfort me. 'Don't cry like that,' said she. 'You can see your children again.'

" 'Don't tell me lies,' I told her. 'They're dead and gone and I'll never see them any more. Where their spirits are, who can tell? I've hung up bits of their clothes on the spirit tree on top of the hill, but how can I think that their tiny spirits, wandering alone and cold, will ever find the clothing I've put out for them? It's my fault because last New Year's day I neglected to tie any scraps of cloth on the spirit tree or to scatter rice beneath it for the spirits, and now they've taken their revenge.' Now turn over and let me massage your back," Do-Ka said.

I turned. It felt good. "Please go on with your story."

"My friend said a strange thing. 'God has your little ones in His care,' she said. 'They're not lonely and lost. Come with me to the house of God next Sunday and learn how you can see your children again.'

" 'When is Sunday, and where's God's house?' I asked.

'I'll come for you on Sunday,' she said. 'It's three days from now.'

"The house of God was just like all our Korean houses, with mud walls, paper doors and windows, thatch roof, and heated floors. But there was a strange person there with green eyes and yellow hair, a high nose, queer clothes, an accent I'd never heard before, and tall, taller than any of our people. This was no ordinary person; this must be God. I listened to find out about my children, but the talk was of something else and I couldn't understand it. I couldn't ask *God* questions, but I decided to go again and learn what I could."

Straightening up, she rubbed her hands together, alternately flexing and extending her fingers to rest them.

"There were no schools when I was a child," she continued, "and I didn't know anything. Can you believe I was ever so foolish as to think Dr. MacMillan was God? When I heard her invite people to bring sick folk next day to be treated, I went to see what God would do. The sick were treated kindly, without paying anything, and several told me they felt much better since taking the medicine they were given. God must be good and would probably need some help to cure all the sick people in Wonsan. I went every day to help God and I learned a lot. Can you believe it was nearly a year before I realized this kindly and skillful healer wasn't God, but a devoted doctor doing His work for Him? That's how stupid I was." She laughed quietly. "Don't you want to go to sleep?"

"Not yet. Please finish your story."

She put her hand on my brow. "The fever's gone down," she said with satisfaction, and sat cross-legged on the floor. "My husband died the next year and when Dr. MacMillan came to Hamheung to begin medical work here, I came with her. For nearly twenty years we worked together, and now she's gone." Her voice quavered. "And you've come in her place. I'll do my best for you."

She leaned forward, her face in her hands, touching the

floor. "Our Father God," she prayed, "all thanks to You for sending missionaries to our dark land to tell us of Your love and mercy and forgiveness, and to heal our bodies and let You heal our souls. Bless this new young doctor and give her health and strength, skill and wisdom for any situation she has to face. Help us all to love and work together so that those who don't know Your love may see it in us and come to know their Father God. Amen."

She rose and tucked me in.

"Sleep in peace. I'll watch the hospital," she said.

The door closed softly and I slept.

-8-

Although it soon became known throughout the countryside that *Maing Pouine's* Hospital was open again, it took longer for Maing Pouine's successor to train a staff and win the confidence of the public.

Soon after the hospital opened, a poorly dressed woman about thirty years of age applied for a job. Since she produced no sons, her husband had abandoned her in favor of another woman and she had to earn her living anyway she could.

"We need someone in the laundry," I told her. "Are you willing to work there?"

"I'll do anything you tell me," she said.

She was a good worker, struggling with the washing by hand in concrete laundry tubs and then hanging it on the line outside in good weather and near the furnace when it rained. If the wind were in the wrong direction, the clean laundry sometimes got grimy again from coal smoke and had to be done over, but the washwoman never complained.

She joined the staff and the ambulatory patients so inclined for morning prayers. Seeing others with Bible and hymn-book, she was determined to learn to read and possess books of her own.

She asked Lee Sunsaing to print the Lord's Prayer and ten

commandments in large clear letters on separate sheets of paper; one on the wall above the washtubs and the other over the ironing board. She asked anyone passing by to teach her one syllable, for Korean is written in syllables rather than in single letters. The next person happening along taught her one more, and in a short time she could read. She bought her own Bible and hymnbook and joined in the singing and reading. It wasn't long before she decided to be a Christian. Kang Do-Ka was happy to teach her and take her to church where she found a gracious fellowship and new friends to comfort her lonely heart.

When her faithless husband's second wife fell sick and was in turn deserted by the man, the washwoman visited the sick woman, brought her to the hospital, had her admitted, and paid the expenses herself. A year later, the second wife again became ill. The laundrywoman once more paid the hospital and after the death of her supplanter adopted the other woman's child. I wondered how many more advanced Christians would have done as much.

As the number of patients increased, so did the work in the laundry, and the laundress requested a helper. She had one to suggest, her nephew, a strong boy, but not too bright. He was a good worker if he had someone to supervise him and she would guarantee that with her supervision he would be satisfactory. They made a good team.

Some months later, as I arrived at the hospital one morning, an indignant Yum Ke-Moon confronted me. His face was red, his hair disheveled, his shirt torn.

"I went to the laundry to look for a missing blanket," he burst out, "and the laundry boy got angry and struck me. When I resisted, the woman came to help her nephew, and we got into a fight. They tore my shirt and bruised my arms and chest. They're not fit to work here and should be dismissed at once."

I assured Yum that I would investigate the matter and, in the meantime, he was to keep away from the laundry and say nothing to the people there.

Next day, after tempers had time to cool, and people to reflect on their conduct, I listened again to Yum's story which was somewhat less lurid than on the previous occasion, but the main facts remained the same.

With a silent prayer for wisdom and patience, I summoned the laundry staff.

"What's this I hear about you and Yum Ke-Moon?" I asked.

"He came into the laundry and accused us of stealing."

"Then what happened?"

"We denied it."

"Then what?"

"He got angry and said it was his business to look after the supplies on his ward, and the best blanket from the private room hadn't come back from the laundry, so one of us should know where it was."

"So then?"

"We got angry too and tried to put him out, and the first thing we knew we were fighting."

"Do you think fighting, shouting, calling bad names, and tearing one another's clothes is proper conduct in a Christian hospital? We're supposed to act in such a way that people will see for themselves that the Christian way of living is better than the old way. What would they think if they saw us fighting among ourselves?"

They hung their heads and didn't reply.

"I'm responsible for the work and conduct in this hospital and I can't have fighting here," I said. "What do you think I should do?"

Again no reply.

"What would you do if you were in my place?"

"There's nothing to do but dismiss us."

"You've worked well for a long time and everybody likes you. I don't want to dismiss anyone for one mistake, but you realize we can't have fighting among the employees. And no one's found the blanket. Can you promise there won't be any more trouble between you and Ke-Moon if you stay?"

"We wouldn't want to promise and then break our word,"

said the woman, "and we're so angry at him we don't know what we'd do if he came to the laundry again. You better dismiss us."

"I'm not dismissing you. If you want to leave I can't stop you, but I'm not dismissing you. I hope you'll promise not to make any more trouble and decide to stay."

"We can't promise. We'll have to go."

Next day they failed to appear and we sent for temporary help in the laundry.

About ten o'clock one evening, several days later, there was a timid knock on my door. It was the laundrywoman and her nephew, she with a potted plant on her head, he carrying a big bundle wrapped in a large square of cotton. After the usual greetings, she presented me with the plant and the boy opened his bundle. There was the missing blanket.

"I'm so ashamed I've no words to express it," said the woman, "I didn't think this boy would do such a thing as take anything that didn't belong to him, but last night I was at his house and saw the blanket. Here it is. Can you forgive us?"

"Of course I forgive you. You confess your fault and bring back the blanket. Now I know you'll not do such a thing again."

There was a long pause. Then, "Is there anyone in our place in the laundry?"

"Just temporarily. We've been keeping your places for you."

"Then we can go back?"

"Come back tomorrow and forgive Yum. I'm sure he'll forgive you. There were faults on both sides since nobody can fight alone."

"Thank you. Thank you. We'll be there."

"That's fine. Now let's have prayer together before you go."

We knelt.

"Loving and merciful Father, we give thanks to Thee for forgiveness and for bringing us together again. Help us to live and work together in peace with everyone and always remember we are Thy children."

Next morning they were on duty. They apologized to Yum and he got his blanket back. They forgave each other and never again was there any trouble between them.

One of my first patients, an elderly Korean gentleman, wearing a high black horsehair hat over his topknot, his long white beard sweeping his chest, walked with dignity into my examining room and extended a hand. "Feel my pulse," he demanded. "What's the sickness?"

He told me nothing of the nature of his complaint and refused any other examination. The traditional Korean doctor, who learned what he knew by apprenticing with a practitioner of ancient Chinese medicine, was accustomed to making diagnoses by feeling the pulse. If I couldn't do the same, obviously I didn't know as much. This wasn't the only such patient I encountered. Many had more faith in these traditional practitioners of Chinese medicine. Some went shopping around to see who would guarantee a cure in the shortest time for the least money. "How many days will it take you to cure me?" was a frequent question. Since I merely undertook to do my best and didn't guarantee a cure within a stated number of days, they often went where the best bargain was promised, sometimes returning later when their money was gone and the condition worse.

Many in need of surgical treatment lacked confidence enough to accept advice and went home to see if they wouldn't get better without treatment. These, too, frequently returned later after much suffering with the condition far advanced.

Others feared the anesthetic. They knew we could put them to sleep, but weren't so sure we could wake them up again. After hearing Lee Sunsaing explain, I wasn't surprised. I told a patient he needed an operation to remove an abdominal tumor and he turned to Lee Sunsaing.

"Does she know anything about our Korean insides?" he inquired anxiously, pointing at me with his chin.

"She knows all about them," Lee replied. "She's looked inside dozens of our people and removed their diseases."

"How can she do that?"

"You'll lie down comfortably on a table and the doctor will cut you open and take out the disease. Then she'll sew you up again and you'll be well."

"But that would hurt terribly. I couldn't endure the pain."

"You won't feel any pain. We'll give you medicine to breathe till you're quite dead, then the doctor will cut out the sickness, and after you're cured, we'll bring you back to life again."

It wasn't unusual for people who had never been in a hospital or known anyone who'd had surgery to hesitate before being killed quite dead in order to be cured. Added to that was the common belief that every time a person had an anesthetic his life would be shortened by five years.

Some came at such a late stage that with any treatment the prospect was poor, sometimes hopeless. If someone died after belated surgical treatment, the family would likely blame the surgeon for causing the death. In risky cases, I explained to the family that had they brought the sick one early the operation could have been done without much danger, but that such a time was already past. Without surgery there was no hope, but at this stage it would be difficult and the risk great. If the family decided to request it and accepted responsibility for the result, I would do my best to save the life of the sick one by operating.

Traditionally the oldest member of the family made the decision. Since the oldest was likely to be the least educated and most distrustful of new ways, he was apt to refuse to let the patient have his one chance for life. If the patient wanted the operation and grandfather said, "no," nothing could be done, the sufferer would be carried home to die.

For five years I never saw an appendix. There were plenty of patients with acute appendicitis, but they never came until after two or more days of the wrong treatment had resulted in serious complications. Sometimes there was a large abscess surrounding a ruptured appendix that had sloughed away completely, or the whole abdomen might be full of pus and all that could be done was to let it out. Though there were no antibiotics—not even sulfa drugs in those days —it was amazing how often such patients recovered after surgical treatment.

Since no family would permit surgery without some member of the household in the operating room to see that the doctor didn't remove some part to make "medicine" out of it, we took the opportunity to teach. When a patient with neglected appendicitis was admitted suffering from peritonitis and likely to die with an abdomen full of pus, we explained before the operation that the appendix had been left so long that it was causing the fever and pain. We said the purgatives the sufferer had been given had made the condition worse. On the abdomen being opened, the smell was often enough to convince the onlooker that we were right. It was even more convincing when the pus was under such pressure that it spouted up like a fountain before streaming to the floor.

Within five years, people from scores of villages throughout South Hamkyung province learned about appendicitis. They came to know that a person with a sudden severe pain in the lower abdomen on the right side should not be given strong purgatives, but should be taken promptly to the hospital. Patients began to come early before complications occurred. Thus, operating on an appendix became a satisfaction instead of a nightmare.

It took longer to overcome the dread of baths during illness. One morning I admitted a young man, who had been ill for more than a year. Dirt was caked on him. Yum Nu-Ka undertook to give him a bed-bath since he was too weak to go in the tub. That afternoon Yum couldn't be found. I finally discovered him bathing the patient.

"Whatever is taking you so long?" I asked.

"I've used seventeen basins of water, and he's not clean yet," explained the attendant.

Such devotion to duty could hardly be reprimanded.

A boy suffering from bone infection had been a patient in the government hospital for fifteen months during which time he hadn't had a bath. Nurses there didn't give baths and patients didn't want them. This boy, with his discharging sores, couldn't be put to soak in the bathtub and it took numerous scrubbings and several days before he was really clean.

Though patients and families were apprehensive at our insistence that everyone admitted should have a bath and put on clean hospital clothes, patients declared they felt refreshed after the ordeal. They certainly smelled better until they put on their own soiled clothes again, often under the clean pajamas provided by the hospital.

A disconcerting experience was to find a practitioner of Chinese medicine treating one of my patients with his medications and methods right in our ward. Neither patient nor practitioner was ever in the least embarrassed when I discovered them. I used to advise the patient to take either my treatment or the practitioner, but not both simultaneously. If he wanted Chinese medicine that was fine with me, but he had to go to the other man's hospital to get it. Most local doctors, modern or native style, had a few hot-floor rooms where they admitted patients though they didn't supply food, nursing service, or other facilities usually associated with hospitals. People felt at home on the hot floors and considered beds cold, comfortless, and risky affairs.

People more than once implored me to treat a sick friend in the government hospital or some private one. This was distressing since the family did not understand my refusal and thought it was due to lack of interest and a desire to help. The few doctors in the city with modern training had no idea of medical ethics as known in the West. Medicine was a business rather than a profession. Doctors were not held in high regard by the public and preferred to be called teacher instead of doctor.

An elderly man with a fracture of both bones above the wrist joint had had the *chim* needles inserted one hundred times in his hand and wrist. This was "to let the bad blood out," according to the native doctor, who, in spite of the obvious deformity, had failed to recognize the fracture. When I saw the unfortunate victim several days later, pus was oozing from each puncture, the hand and arm were greatly swollen, the pain severe, and the infection introduced by the dirty needle had entered the bloodstream. In spite of all we could do, the man nearly lost his life and had a permanently useless right hand.

We always had prayer in the operating room before the anesthetic was started. During specially difficult operations, Kang Do-Ka and the hospital evangelist often remained outside the door praying for surgeon and patient. Even those who were not Christians sometimes told me they came to our hospital because they knew we had prayer before operating, and emergency surgery performed under unfavorable conditions was successful in a gratifying number of cases.

Besides practitioners of *chim* and *doom,* who used dried lizards and deerhorn, there was still another practitioner of the healing art—the *mudang* (sorceress) who specialized in exorcising evil spirits that were believed to cause disease. These women spent as much time as the family could afford in singing, shouting, dancing, beating cymbals, and gyrating to drive the spirit out. They raised such a racket and would keep it up so long, that only very dull or stupid spirits lingered around. If the patient could endure the pandemonium, he had a good chance of recovery, in spite of, rather than because of, the exorcism.

Home remedies could also be as disastrous. A doctor from the Methodist Mission Hospital in Wonsan told me of a woman who was brought to him after her husband had shot off a gun beside her to frighten away the spirit that was believed to be causing mental illness. There was then plenty of room for it to escape for the man had blown off the side of his wife's head.

Fractured limbs, I found, were generally bound up with neat splints made of bark stripped from trees. However, the splints were invariably too short to control the broken bone adequately, and when the inevitable swelling occurred, they became too tight, causing severe pain, cutting into the flesh, and interfering with circulation. If the splint was left on too long, as was usually the case, gangrene resulted.

The usual home treatment of abscesses and ulcers was to apply a gummy black substance, insoluble in any fluid we ever tried, and almost impossible to remove. This prevented the discharge from escaping and promoted its burrowing into the tissues.

Favorite applications to inflamed or injured parts was a handful of dusty cobwebs, road dust, or barnyard manure kept in place by bandages over several layers of cabbage leaves. Serious infection often followed. I was amazed that tetanus (lockjaw) was not more frequent. I rarely saw it except in newborn babies. Here the bacilli were introduced by cutting the umbilical cord with dirty kitchen scissors or sawing it with a blade of coarse grass. Obviously, Korean patients who survived the early years developed considerable immunity to various infections.

One night, after I had moved from the hospital and was living in a new house built for the mission women, a commotion in the garden awakened me. Two men were standing under a big acacia tree outside my window and a third was in the upper branches.

"Whatever are you doing in our garden this time of night?" I demanded.

"Trying to catch a magpie," one replied.

"What do you want with a magpie? And where is there any such custom as going into someone's garden in the middle of the night and making all this disturbance?"

"A friend has a bad sore on his neck and can't sleep for the pain. We need a magpie to split open and put on his neck, and we saw a nest in this tree. We're trying to catch the bird."

"Wouldn't it be better to take your friend to the hospital and have the doctor treat him?"

"We've no money to go to the hospital and a magpie's a sure cure."

The noise they made frightened the birds away, and I

never learned the fate of the man with the carbuncle.

The torture meted out by traveling old crones who professed to cure women suffering from neglected complications of childbirth was barbarous. Subjected to unwise treatment by ignorant midwives, these women were expected to get up as soon as the baby was born and go to the river to wash the soiled clothing. The heavy uterus often sagged down into the dilated birth canal which resulted in permanent displacement which in turn led to other difficulties. Some victims could neither sit nor walk comfortably. Too modest or too impecunious to go to a hospital, they patronized the ignorant creatures who preyed upon their misfortune. Usually, only after much suffering and further complications, did they finally seek sensible treatment.

"What is your complaint?" I asked a wretched looking woman in the clinic, though from the smell I already suspected.

Embarrassed she hung her head. "My clothes are always wet," she whispered.

"How long have you been like this? What caused it?"

"After my last baby was born something seemed to come out. I couldn't sit or walk comfortably, but I had to look after the children and the house. A woman who said she could cure me took the kitchen knife and cut off something. Ever since then my clothes are wet all the time and my feet soaking in my rubber shoes. The smell is so bad they won't let me sleep in the house. I can sleep outside in the summer but I'm worn out washing my clothes and bedding every day, and now it'll soon be winter. How can I sleep outside in the winter? I'll die if I have to go on like this. *Sal lyo chusio.*"

The whole front wall of her bladder was gone and the remaining tissues so contracted it was impossible to close the bladder completely. Other cases where the damage was less extensive could be cured, though it often took more than one operation. All I could do in this case was to direct the urine into the lower bowel and close off the front passage completely. This gave control, but after such treatment women could no longer have children, and their husbands seldom wanted them.

Another method of the quacks was to wind a strong cord firmly around the displaced parts to cut off the blood supply until the flesh sloughed away. The suffering endured while this was taking place can hardly be imagined. Though the prolapse was often cured, other problems, equally distressing, usually followed.

Others packed the birth passage with rags soaked in kerosene and set them on fire. The contraction of the scar following this terrible treatment effectively cured the descent of the parts, but often resulted in serious, even fatal, complications.

If pregnancy didn't occur, the wife was likely to be cast off as useless. If it did, the child could not be born through the contracted passage and mother and child might—and often did—die in childbirth. I dreaded to see a maternity case come to the hospital since normal ones seldom came, and complicated ones appeared only after days of suffering with the child dead and the mother exhausted and usually infected from the misguided efforts of an untrained midwife trying to deliver the child.

Home cure for snakebite consisted of tying off the limb well above the bite. A switch of a woman's long, heavy hair was used for this purpose. This was intended to prevent the real or imagined poison—for Korea has few venomous snakes—from entering the general circulation. This it did, but the switch was invariably left on for hours until the part below the tie off became gangrenous from lack of circulation.

One of my early patients was a young woman who had been given this treatment for snakebite three months before. No one knew whether the snake was poisonous or not, and it probably wasn't. From three inches below the knee where the switch had been applied the flesh was black, shriveled, and gangrenous. It had separated from the living flesh above, which left a space of three inches between them. The stench was almost unbearable.

I explained that the lower leg was dead and should be removed to get rid of the decayed flesh and permit the woman to get a useful artificial leg.

The husband insisted that I put the leg back together again. If I would do that he was sure it would soon heal and be well again. When I said that was impossible, they left with some hard words for a doctor who would take off an unfortunate person's leg without even trying to put it together, when anyone could see that was what was needed.

Everyday, and often night, was filled with work.

In addition to emergency cases requiring attention, nights were sometimes interrupted by shouting, screaming, and name calling with occasional sounds of blows from nearby houses. Quarrels seemed to be a nightly occurrence and often developed into wife and child beating accompanied by the screams of the victims. My indignation was roused almost to the point of interference. Knowing that to meddle in family affairs would turn both family and community against the outsider and do nothing to help the domestic situation, I kept from any such ill-advised action.

I avoided operating at night as much as possible due to the uncertainty of the electric power from our own small generator, and later from the city generator. After ten at night, when the generator shut down, light for the wards was supplied by candles and small oil lamps. The illumination from city power was feeble and often failed altogether. In my bedroom in the hospital I had a large kerosene oil lamp with a circular wick that gave a good light for reading, but it couldn't readily be carried around. The tall glass chimney fitted with some difficulty into a sort of frame and the frame and chimney had to be removed together.

Then an emergency case arrived that required immediate surgery. Because of complications, the operation was difficult and time consuming, and at a critical stage the electric lights flickered and died.

"Get the lamp from my room as quickly as possible," I told the night orderly. After fumbling with my door key for much longer than seemed necessary, he finally got the door open and brought the lamp. Before I could warn him, he pulled the chimney out of the frame, lighted the wick, and couldn't get the chimney back in place.

An open flame in the presence of ether is likely to cause an explosion, so the nurse giving anesthetic switched to chloroform. After what seemed a long time, the orderly got the chimney in place and to my great relief I found the patient in a satisfactory condition. As I resumed the operation, the lights came on again. A sigh of relief went up from the operating-room staff and the orderly blew out the lamp. The power promptly went off again and remained off the rest of the night. The orderly relighted the lamp. I completed the operation, and the patient was returned to the ward in good condition, despite the nerve-racking experience of the surgeon.

After flashlights became available, we used them in the wards at night and in the operating room when the power failed. They had the double advantage of being safe in the presence of ether and of directing light into the wound where it was needed.

About this time, the arrival of a teacher for missionary children gave me much cheer. It had been lonely living in the hospital away from anyone who spoke my language.

Florence Hall, from Calgary in Alberta, Canada, was a slender, blue-eyed young woman with blonde hair, a cheery smile, and a well-developed sense of humor. She came to live in an unoccupied room next to mine in the hospital, and we fixed up another for a common living room. She was about my age and it was delightful to have someone to talk to in English who shared a similar background. In late afternoon, when our tasks were over, we often climbed Dragon Hill or strolled in the city streets followed by crowds of children crying out, "Goot pyee, Goot pyee," their way of pronouncing goodbye, the only words of English they knew. As they used it, it was a word of greeting.

Miss Hall was a light sleeper and the barking of the neighborhood dogs often kept her awake at night. Sometimes on returning to my room after a call to the wards, I met Miss Hall dragging the mattress from her bed across the corridor to a vacant room at the back of the building, away from the noise at the front. Thinking that the noisy mongrels would not be highly valued and might be purchased and disposed of, she found to her surprise that not one was for sale.

"Why can't I buy them?" she asked Lee Sunsaing who was doing the bargaining for her.

"They're not fat this time of year," he said. "In another couple of months they'll be fat and worth more. No one eats dog this time of year."

An eagerly anticipated event was the arrival from Toronto, Canada, of a trained nurse, Miss Viola Cardwell. Viola was a tall, brown-haired girl whose gray eyes and friendly smile soon won the hearts of all who knew her. She carried herself well and had a penchant for smart clothes. Her capable hands and strong sense of responsibility indicated her fitness for her task as superintendent of nursing and instructor of nursing attendants in Cheihei Hospital. I could hardly wait for her to complete her course at language school and come to join me in the hospital.

Then one of our group who had been in poor health for some time became pregnant. Her overworked and weakened kidneys could not take the strain, and gradually failed. Finally, she became so swollen and heavy she couldn't move in bed. We had to summon Viola from language school in Seoul to come and nurse her.

The baby came prematurely, but too late for the mother whose kidneys could no longer function. About midnight of the second day after delivery, it was obvious the end was not far off. We were both watching her when the lights flickered and went out.

We waited.

A flicker again, and the light slowly came on.

The figure on the bed lay inert and motionless except for heavy breathing that became more and more labored, with the intervals between breaths longer and longer.

"Better call the others," I said at last. "They want to be here so the husband won't be alone when his wife leaves us."

She had said farewell to us in the morning and requested to be buried in her wedding dress. Viola and I looked at one another. At her marriage she had weighed ninety-five pounds.

At midday she became unconscious. There was nothing we could do but watch and wait.

The other adults in the little foreign community soon arrived. Silently they wrung the hand of the sorrowing husband and stood back in quiet sympathy.

The breathing of the dying woman became louder and more difficult. Viola bent over her wiping cold sweat from the unconscious face, while I stood on the other side of the bed with fingers on the weakening pulse that was missing more and more beats.

As we watched, the lights flickered and went out. Another labored breath broke the stillness. I felt a few more pulsations, and again silence pervaded the room. The light flickered and came on dimly. Another breath and the light died away. No one moved or spoke.

Once more for a few seconds the light flashed on accompanied by another stertorous breath and a few more heartbeats, then silence and darkness. Would there be another breath, or was our friend gone? We waited, hushed, listening intently.

For the fourth time the light flickered—flickered—and died away. As it did so, the woman on the bed drew a last feeble breath and her tired heart gave up the struggle. No sound broke the somber stillness. No one moved.

In that solemn moment, the quiet room seemed filled with a mysterious presence as though angel wings were hovering near to bear away the weary spirit to the realm where there is no night nor darkness for the glory of God gives it light.

-9-

Every Sunday we newcomers went to the nearest church, across the road from the hospital. This was the first church built in the province. It was a large L-shaped building of wood framework, whitewashed mud walls and ceiling, glass windows, a polished wood floor, and a tiled roof gracefully upswept, Korean style, at the corners. About two hundred people sat cross-legged on the floor, a partition at the angle separating the men and women. No one on one side could see anyone on the other. The minister standing in the corner in between could see and be seen by all.

Kim *Moksa,* Pastor, conducted the service with dignity. Though as new arrivals we didn't understand a word, the music was familiar and there was no mistaking the heartiness of the singing or the earnestness of the prayers and sermon.

At the end of the service, pastor and people gave us a welcome that warmed our hearts. Though the language was strange and much else unfamiliar, the people made us feel surrounded by friends and goodwill.

We attended the evening service too, and I still remember the long row of small black heads resting on the edge of the low platform where the pulpit stood. Children sat at the front and one after another heads went down as the little ones asleep, even after their mothers gathered them up at the close of the service and carried them home on their backs.

This church was built from the efforts of the Reverend Duncan McRae, the first foreigner to live in the conservative city of Hamheung. When they first arrived, Mr. and Mrs. McRae were stoned and driven out. Not long after, they returned again at night, in sedan chairs. Their arrival passed unnoticed and they were allowed to remain.

A few years later, when there were enough Christians to undertake the building of a church, they banded together to do the work. They went to the nearest mountain, cut trees, and, hitching themselves to the logs, dragged them down to the building site at the foot of Dragon Hill. As this place was believed to be haunted, no one objected to the Christians using it. Here they squared the timber, sawed it into posts, planks, and boards, and using whole tree trunks for the corners, they erected the first church.

When we arrived, there was a second church in the downtown area. This was known as the lower church, and the first was called the upper church. The lower church was a two-story red brick building with a gallery. Although it had no architectural beauty, it was one of the largest buildings in Hamheung and the congregation who planned, financed, and built it were proud of it. Ethel McEachern attended this church and for two or three years I went with her. It was a mile walk from our quarters near the hospital, the girl's school, and the upper church. On dark nights, we carried kerosene lanterns through the unlighted streets, but most of the congregation had paper lanterns, a candle burning brightly in each as it dangled on the end of a hand-held stick. These little lights, flickering and bobbing in the dark streets, made a pretty sight.

The evening service began at dark—six o'clock in the winter but in the long summer evenings it might begin sometime past nine. As many had no watch or clock, people told time from the sun and the church bell.

Inside the separate entrances for men and women were

shelves for shoes. No Korean would be crude enough to wear shoes inside a building where people sat on the floor. In railway stations, post offices, and public buildings where people wore shoes, they considered the floor the same as the ground outside and made no effort to keep it clean or tidy. But church and house floors were spotless. Unfortunately, the straw matting on the floor was the dwelling place of numerous fleas who had no objection whatever to the flavor of foreign blood.

The two city churches had pastors, but village congregations couldn't afford to pay a pastor enough to live on and elders or deacons conducted the services and led the Christian worship there.

Becoming a church member involved more than standing up and making a vow to be faithful to Christ. If a new believer was illiterate, he first had to learn to read; then he became an inquirer and was instructed for six months, after which he was examined. If he did well, he entered the second stage. Before being baptized, he had to show an understanding of the Christian faith and prove he had preached to others. To some this examination was quite an ordeal.

One old woman was worried that she mightn't pass and her daughter-in-law was helping her prepare for it.

"If they ask you, 'Why did Jesus die?' " instructed the daughter-in-law, "you must say, 'He died for my sins.' "

The day came. The question was asked, and the old lady triumphantly replied, "He died for my daughter-in-law's sins."

On baptism day, a long row of men and women in shining white clothing sat at the front of the church. One by one, as their names were called, each stood up in his place. When all were standing, the pastor asked if they had decided to believe and follow Jesus. They replied, "Yes." The pastor next asked, "Have you led anyone else to Jesus?" Here and there throughout the church one and another rose and said: "He brought me." "She brought me."

After the group was baptized, the sacrament of the Lord's

Supper was celebrated with somewhat less dignity and reverence than usual in the West, but with deep meaning for those who partook.

By this time, the objection to women singing in church choirs had been overcome and there were choirs in both churches. Sometimes, the young singers brought their music to our house and asked Ethel to play and teach them new hymns and songs. One night they asked her to play the rousing old college song, "The bulldog on the bank and the bullfrog in the pool! The bulldog call'd the bullfrog a green old water fool." She obliged and everyone went home happy.

At church the following Sunday the pastor announced special music by the choir. The leader came across to the women's side and asked Ethel to play. The music placed before her on the organ was that of "The Bulldog on the Bank." Surely, she thought, they must be going to sing other words to that tune, something more appropriate to a church service. Everyone was waiting. With some misgiving, she began to play the rollicking song. The choir sang with gusto a literal translation. The congregation apparently noticed nothing incongruous, but the idea of the dignified and proper Ethel playing that music to those words for an anthem in church was almost too much for me.

To many Korean Christians, God seems more real and near than to most Western churchgoers. Former animistic beliefs no doubt have something to do with this. Animism teaches that the world is filled with spirits inhabiting every tree, rock, mountain, house, river, and every other object. Women, especially, lived in fear of the spirits, most of whom were believed to be malevolent and likely to bring trouble on people unless kept propitiated. These spirits were thought to be the cause of sickness, crop failures, and other disasters.

The word for God in Korean is *Hananim,* the Great One, the supreme or Great One, the One like whom there is no other, the Great Spirit. There was a general belief that the Great Spirit began the world and then went about His own affairs, paying no attention to the puny humans who were left to fend for themselves. Christians, believing that God loves and cares for them, lost their fear of the spirits. With the Great Spirit on their side, what harm could the lesser ones do?

Once as Kang Do-Ka and I were walking past the upper church she began to laugh. "Do you know," she said, "this was the worst place in Hamheung for bad spirits. Nobody ever came here alone even in the daytime and at night it was fearsome to pass here in groups, but since the church was built, the spirits have all left. They won't stay near a church and now anyone can go here alone, even at night."

Even a staunch Christian like Do-Ka could not altogether shake off the old beliefs that had so dominated her life, but she was no longer afraid.

A devoted evangelist told of an experience in his youth before anyone in his village had heard the Gospel. He was sent to take a message to some one in a village at the other side of the mountain from his home. News that a tiger had been recently seen on the mountain made him hurry to reach the other village before dark. By the time he got to the summit, the sun was getting low in the sky, but afraid of the tiger as he was, he was still more afraid of the spirit of the mountain. He didn't dare start down without paying his respects to the mountain spirit—a spirit more fearsome than a tiger—by placing a stone on the cairn erected in its honor.

One of the blessings Christ brought to His followers was the release from such superstitious fears. Many thus blessed were eager to pass on the message to others.

Not content with merely preaching, practically every congregation used the church building as a kindergarten by day and a night school in the evenings. The young people of the church served without remuneration as teachers. Since there were schools enough for only twenty percent of the children of the country (and probably not more than five percent of girls) these church schools filled an important place in the community.

The local YMCA with an enlightened and progressive Korean elder as general secretary conducted both day and night schools for boys.

In order that Christian women might be trained and organized for more effective church and community service, Miss Louise McCully of Wonsan started and promoted among the churches a women's evangelistic society. Few of the members had been to school and could read with difficulty if at all, while their writing was likely to be limited to signing their names if they had any. Most had never in their lives attended any kind of meeting except a regular church worship service.

According to custom, younger women, even though better qualified educationally, would not accept office and conduct meetings if there were older women there to do it.

Ethel McEachran was helping the women's group in the lower church and Mrs. McRae in the upper one, and I began assisting in a small church across the river.

The church was a mud building with paper doors and windows, a thatch roof, and straw matting on the mud floor. When I arrived for the morning service, fifty or sixty Sunday school children taught by schoolboys would be leaving to make room for the adults, while the dust raised by their active feet was almost enough to choke anybody. Someone would open all the windows and any heat that had accumulated would escape with the dust.

The leader, an uneducated elder, would then teach the Sunday school Bible lesson for an hour to the adults before the worship service that he also conducted. The schoolboys in the congregation had more education than he, but he did his best and was always treated with respect. People loved to sing and though musicians might not consider it music, they raised "a joyful noise unto the Lord," and doubtless He accepted it as such.

Edna McLellan on returning from a country trip among the churches was telling of a new church in the mountains. She said they had a choir.

"A choir! Already!" I exclaimed. "Do they sing the four parts?"

"Yes," said Edna, smiling, "Twenty-four."

When the women's society was organized, only two of about twenty members could read. One of these became secretary, the other treasurer. They appointed me president as none of the others knew how to conduct a meeting. They decided to let their contributions accumulate until they had enough to do to contribute toward helping pay the salary of a pastor whom the church hoped to acquire. At the end of the first year, someone asked how we should celebrate the anniversary of the founding of our society.

"We have money," said another. "We might have a feast."

Before this idea took spark, I hastened to ask, "Do we want to spend our money on ourselves? Do you remember what we raised it for? How would it be if we celebrate our birthday as a society by making a contribution to the funds of the church? We might let people know about our society too. Even in our own congregation the men don't know what we are doing, and other women might join if they knew."

"That would be fine," said the secretary, "but would women be allowed to speak in church?"

After some discussion, we appointed a committee to ask the elder's permission to tell about the work of the Women's Evangelistic Society at one of the regular church services.

The elder replied to this request that of course it wouldn't do for a woman to speak at the morning service and at night a man would have to preach first, but if one of the women wanted to speak after the regular service was over, it probably wouldn't do any harm.

On receiving this grudging permission, we arranged for an educated woman, who was a good speaker, to come from one of the city churches to give a report of the first annual meeting of the national Women's Evangelistic Society of the Korean Presbyterian Church. There was a big turnout of non-Christians as well as church people to hear what a woman would say in church. Men were amazed that a woman could speak so well and women were proud.

As the church across the river grew in numbers, it finally

felt able to support a woman evangelist whose family responsibilities would be less than those of a pastor. She could live in a room instead of a house, and live on what the church could manage to pay.

Most women evangelists were widows or deserted wives, the only ones available for study and full-time work outside the home. Though most had little general education, they were strong in the faith, full of enthusiasm, and had been well grounded in the scriptures by the McCully sisters in the Wonsan Bible School. These women evangelists met women in and outside the church on their own level. In work among women, they were more effective than ministers, especially the more educated ones about whom his flock boasted. "He's just wonderful," one said. "He's so learned we can't understand him at all."

We gave our new woman evangelist, Kim Wha-Soon, a warm welcome. The society members took her around and introduced her to the church people, the poor, and those in trouble of any kind. Wha-Soon was middle-aged, short, stout, plain of face, talkative, and energetic. Her genuine feeling of friendship toward everyone made her popular and trusted. Her preaching and exhortations were accompanied by obvious interest and concern and the little church began to grow more rapidly.

About this time, the Christian community in and around Hamheung, desiring to call public attention to the church and its works decided to have a parade through the city. They secured permission and made plans.

The November day proved cold and blustery, dust blowing about in clouds and getting in eyes, noses, and mouths, but that deterred no one. It was too great an occasion.

The Yungsaing Boys' Academy band led the parade followed by five hundred boys and their teachers. Next came seven hundred girls and their teachers from primary, middle, and high-school departments of the Yungsaing Girls' School. After them marched the YMCA and their day and night schools. The lower church followed with its Sunday and day schools, five hundred strong. The upper church followed the little group of missionaries, and as many of the hospital staff as could leave the patients—the nurses conspicuous in their uniforms, caps, and blue capes lined with red. The procession was so long that no one could see all of it at once. Those in the middle couldn't hear the band, while those near the end couldn't hear the middle. As a result, each section followed its own leader and sang its own choice of hymns of joy and praise.

The city looked, listened, and was impressed, not only at the total number of Christians but at the schools, hospital staff, and at the orderliness, enthusiasm, and happiness of the paraders.

-10-

The thirty beds in the main hospital were well utilized. Ten others in a small isolation building beside the main hospital were used occasionally and proved to be a constant source of worry. The only other isolation accommodation in Hamheung was the government pesthouse where there were no beds, no nurses, infrequent visits by a doctor, and little in the way of patient facilities. It was commonly said that no one taken there ever came out alive. The mission thought we should provide better service than that. However, people failed to understand why isolation was necessary, and when anyone was sick all his friends felt they must go to see him.

The law required the hospital to report to the police any infectious disease diagnosed and all admissions and discharges of such patients. We had to get police permission to discharge anyone with an infectious disease. Since most such patients were children, that meant the mother or grandmother had to be admitted too, and since they were uncontrollable, we had our problems. A grandmother with a small diphtheria patient on her back would, in spite of all the nurses could say or do, visit the other patients in their rooms, which broke isolation and spread the disease we were trying to control. If reprimanded, she would take the child and go home. Then we would be in trouble with the police for letting the patient go without their permission. That they sneaked away at night without the doctor knowing was no excuse. This happened so often the patients were seldom helped and the hospital was often in trouble with the police.

I thought it would be better to give up the futile struggle to isolate acute infectious cases and instead provide care for some of the many tuberculosis patients for whom there was no provision anywhere else. The mission agreed and the police finally gave us permission to accept tuberculosis patients instead of ones with acute infections.

A diagnosis of tuberculosis was generally regarded as a sentence of death. Since doctors knew of no one who had recovered, they made no effort to treat such patients. Medical students were left in ignorance regarding the disease. People sometimes committed suicide rather than endure what they believed would be a long drawn-out fatal illness. Though we could not admit many in our small building, we tried to do what we could to help some and inspire hope in others.

At that time there was no drug of any value for treatment, though much could be done to improve the general condition of the patient and relieve distressing symptoms. Rest, fresh air, and nourishing food were the mainstays of treatment. Rest was considered so important that rest hours were definitely prescribed and strictly adhered to. Patients were expected to relax and sleep during afternoon rest hours. This was difficult for Korean patients to understand since they were accustomed to being treated with medicine by the bowlful—the worse the taste the more efficacious it was believed to be. But better still, a large syringeful of fluid shot directly into the bloodstream. Before admitting anyone, I took time to explain the method of treatment, the long time necessary for recovery, and the necessity for cooperation from the patient.

I tried to admit only patients with a reasonable prospect of improvement and intelligence enough to follow the rules, since, if our patients died like others, no one would have cause for hope.

Some, because they didn't feel better in a few days, became discouraged and left, but most of our picked patients cooperated well and recovered. As our staff had had no training in the care of the tuberculous, I undertook that work myself.

Before the isolation building was converted into a tiny tuberculosis sanatorium, one of my first tuberculous patients, was Lee Choon-Chul or Alexander, Dr. Martin's capable interpreter in Yongjung, now a medical student at Severance Medical College. A sudden lung hemorrhage alarmed him greatly. On being told he had tuberculosis—that fatal disease—he left college and went to the Diamond Mountains to rest, but there was no one there to advise or help him.

Much discouraged, he wrote me of his condition. I sent for him and gave him a bed on the veranda in the fresh air, apart from those in the wards. For three months, I spent most of my spare time trying to encourage Choon-Chul by telling him of people I knew who had recovered from the dreaded disease and lived useful lives. At first he scarcely seemed to listen, but I persisted.

"Choon-Chul," I said one day after he had been with us some weeks, "I know you believe in God. Do you think He loves you?"

"Yes, I believe He does, but why has He let this illness come to me?"

"What happens to us in this life doesn't matter as much as how we face up to it. You've probably been crying to God to cure you, but you don't really believe He will or you'd eat your rice and sleep in peace at night instead of refusing food and tossing and worrying the way you do."

He didn't reply.

"Choon-Chul," I said, "I believe the day will come when you'll think this illness that now fills you with despair was a blessing to you."

"That's hard to believe."

"I think so, just the same."

Soon after he realized he was improving he became cheerful, ate, and slept better, and began to make real progress. When he left to return to medical college he reminded me of this conversation and said I had been right. He graduated the top student in his class and won the gold medal.

Among the early patients in our small sanatorium was a seventeen-year-old boy whose widowed mother brought him from a remote mountain village. He had been to school and was intelligent and cooperative, but his mother was not only ignorant, but, unlike most Korean women, loud, rough, domineering, and determined to have her own way. I explained at length the kind of treatment we gave, the necessity for rest and quiet, and the full cooperation of patient and relatives that would be necessary for a good result. Both the boy and his mother agreed to comply with the rules and cooperate in every way with the treatment.

I admitted the lad and all went well until afternoon rest hours from two till four o'clock, when visitors had to leave and patients were expected to rest quietly and if possible sleep. The mother refused to leave. When the nurse asked her to go for two hours, she became angry, shouting that she'd never been separated from her son for one hour and had no intention of leaving him now. She shouted and stormed while other patients were ringing their bells and asking for quiet so they could sleep. Finally, after persuasion failed, Yum Nu-Ka and I took her by the arm, walked her down the corridor, and out the door which we locked behind her.

For the whole rest period she marched up and down on the landing outside the door shouting, yelling, screaming, cursing, pounding on the door, and abusing the hospital. No patient in either building had any rest that day.

That evening she repeated the performance. I was at my wit's end. If we gave in to her, the other patients' relatives would insist on staying too and the whole plan of rest hours so important for treatment would go by the board. So I hardened my heart hoping I was doing the right thing and that once she realized the hospital routine would have to be followed, she might cooperate.

When I went home at midnight she was still going strong, yelling, screeching, shouting curses and imprecations on the hospital and all connected with it. I didn't sleep much. Neither did anyone in the hospital. Was I doing the right thing? At five in the morning my telephone rang. She had dislocated her jaw.

"Thank the Lord!" I exclaimed fervently, and took my time dressing and walking over to the hospital. The Lord had delivered her into my hands, and who was I not to cooperate with the Almighty? A little reflection on her conduct and its result wouldn't do her any harm.

There she was, still marching up and down before the hospital door, incoherent but still shouting. When she saw me coming, she ran to meet me pointing to her fallen jaw and signing to me imperiously to help her.

I backed off and bargained with her. If she would cease her noise and follow the hospital rules which were for the benefit of the patients and part of the treatment, I would reduce the dislocation. But not until she promised and showed evidence of her good faith by stopping the disturbance. I felt mean taking her at such a disadvantage, but what else could I do? She agreed to stop the racket, and I reduced the dislocation. Since she couldn't endure being separated from her son even for an hour, she took him home that day. Without treatment, he was no doubt permanently separated from her within a year.

Fortunately, most of our patients cooperated well and so many recovered that within a few years people all over the province heard of someone who had recovered from tuberculosis and hope began to replace despair.

Considerably later we acquired a portable x-ray machine and, small as it was, it was most helpful in chest work. I ran it myself until I could train one of the nurses as an x-ray technician.

Later still, when local compression of the lung by introducing air between it and the chest wall was introduced as treatment in suitable cases, I made my own pneumothorax apparatus. It cost about three dollars instead of the sixty that the cheapest machine would have cost, and it worked just as well.

A further development in the treatment of tuberculosis was to compress the lung in appropriate cases by collapsing the chest wall over the affected area. This was a formidable operation involving the removal of several ribs on one side, sometimes on both, and was done only as a last resort in advanced cases, usually to close a chronic cavity in the lung. As long as a cavity remained open, the disease was likely to spread.

I had never seen the operation done, but I bought and studied the latest books on tuberculosis and undertook the operation on a young man who, after several years of treatment, still had a large cavity in his lung. Some years after the operation, he was living and able to work.

Not all tuberculous patients had such satisfactory results.

Dr. Hong, my first medical colleague, had gone to Canada to study tuberculosis and on returning set up as the first specialist in chest diseases in that part of Korea. From him, I heard the history of a patient who came to me as a last resort.

This man was a big burly policeman who developed tuberculous pleurisy and went to Dr. Hong for treatment. The doctor gave him something to relieve the pain and explained carefully that the treatment would take some months and cure depended on the patient's following the doctor's instructions and resting until the disease was under control. When the man wasn't cured in three days, he took the advice of his friends who told him he was getting weak lying around resting. He should instead get up at daybreak, climb Dragon Hill, and exercise his weak lungs by shouting as loud as he could, waving his arms vigorously at the same time. He did this for a few days but felt so much worse he couldn't continue.

Since Dr. Hong hadn't cured him he went to another doctor, and complained of shortness of breath. This doctor drew off a moderate amount of clear fluid from the chest, but he was still too sick and weak to climb the hill.

Obviously the second doctor was no good either and the man went to a third. By this time the fluid had become infected and the third doctor drew off pus. Later, a fourth doctor made an incision between the ribs to let the pus drain away. Then the tuberculosis infection became mixed with other organisms—a much worse condition. Pus continued to leak from the incision while the patient became progressively weaker.

Since doctors hadn't cured him, he resorted to self-treatment. To keep the incision open, he inserted several fine rootlets from a tree. When one day they slipped inside the chest he came to me to have them removed.

Though I tried to keep up-to-date with the treatment of tuberculosis, none of my books gave any instructions on how to remove tree roots from the chest cavity.

Placing the man on his sound side on the operating table, I injected a local anesthetic, enlarged the opening, and looked inside. Though the lung had been collapsed for weeks, I couldn't see the roots which were lying in a sort of trough next to the spine and behind the lung. I poured in a large amount of sterile saline solution and the roots floated up near the incision where I could grasp them with forceps. I removed a dozen rootlets fifteen inches long.

How to treat the man from then on was no problem as he immediately took himself off for more self-treatment. He died a few months later. No doctor can do much for such a patient.

Though I began treating tuberculosis patients out of necessity, my chief satisfaction was in surgery—difficult though it often was. At first I had no other doctor to consult with or assist me. Complications were frequent. Neither oxygen nor blood for tranfusions were available. We had no suction apparatus or x-ray equipment.

When spinal anesthesia came into use, I adopted it in suitable cases. I found it a great help since some patients who refused a general anesthetic were willing to have a spinal. In such cases, I gave the anesthetic myself, then scrubbed and did the operation with Nurse Woo assisting and Lee Sunsaing watching the patient's blood pressure and respiration.

Complications were often due to parasites. Almost every patient had at least one variety. Many had two, and some as many as five different kinds of parasite. Operations on the intestinal tract were frequently complicated by the presence of these intruders. Once during such an operation, a loop of tapeworm appeared in an incision in the bowel. I pulled on the loop gently until thirty feet of worm lay on the floor.

Roundworms were more common and caused more trouble. Sometimes masses of them formed veritable balls of squirming intertwined worms which acted as a foreign body. In an attempt to get rid of it, the intestine clamped down causing severe pain and obstruction that was difficult to distinguish from causes requiring surgical intervention. Several times I operated on a patient with apparent acute intestinal obstruction only to find a mass of tangled worms with the intestine tightly contracted above it causing complete obstruction.

To try to remove the mass of worms was perilous because more worms in other parts of the bowel, irritated by the anesthetic, would travel about and might penetrate the incision in the intestine and carry infection into the abdominal cavity. To leave them was risky, but it was as dangerous to give the toxic drug necessary to evacuate the worms to a patient recovering from an anesthetic. If nothing was done, the obstruction might continue with fatal results. I tried all methods but there were worrisome hours and days for doctor and patient.

Late cases of obstruction, with the patient seriously ill, and the distended bowel above the obstruction full of highly toxic material used to be treated by draining off the toxic contents through a large tube inserted into the bowel. The hope was that the patient's condition would improve sufficiently so that an operation for the relief of the obstruction could then be safely undertaken. In my experience, the drainage tube was soon blocked with worms and many of these cases ended fatally. Fortunately, better methods of treatment are available now.

One experience with the traveling propensities of roundworms followed an abdominal operation in which the intestine was not involved. Though the surgery was completed satisfactorily the patient had a stormy convalescence for which I couldn't account. On the third postoperative day, on inspecting the wound, I discovered a healthy looking specimen of roundworm that, either desiring a change of residence or the experience of travel, had made its way through the intestinal wall and the abdominal incision. Its adventure ended there. Henceforth, the patient made an uneventful recovery.

These worms sometimes entered the appendix where, lacking room to turn around, and with no capacity to back out, attempted to push their way through the tip. This caused pain and other symptoms difficult to distinguish from early appendicitis. At surgery, appendix and worm would be removed together.

I once found a roundworm seized with wanderlust residing in the duct between the ovary and uterus. It didn't seem to be causing any inconvenience to its host but, since such uninvited guests are potential causes of trouble, I dragged it unceremoniously from its lair and it met its fate in the cold world.

I can never forget a seven-year-old girl whose mother brought her for treatment after a long illness, the cause of which had defied diagnosis by several doctors. The child was so weak and ill that recovery seemed most unlikely. I told the mother there was little hope. I was eager to find the cause of the trouble and explained to the mother that if I couldn't make a diagnosis and the child died, it might help to understand a similar case later if we could do an autopsy. Surprisingly the mother agreed to this, partly no doubt because we undertook to do what we could for the child free of charge.

The child had many roundworms, and her condition was so poor that I didn't think it safe to give the usual dose of the toxic medicine necessary to eliminate the parasites. I gave what I thought the patient could tolerate. She got rid of about five hundred worms, but her condition failed to improve. We gave her extra nourishment and a few days later another dose of medicine to expel the remaining worms. Approximately another three hundred were evacuated. A few days later, the child died.

At the autopsy, nearly one hundred living worms were found in the stomach and intestine. Several had ascended the liver ducts and perforated the organ. Thirteen were found impacted in the main bile duct obstructing it completely. Three perforations in the large bowel led into abdominal abscess cavities containing more worms. No wonder the child died. The wonder is that she survived so long.

These worms sometimes go far afield, even entering the bronchial tubes. I once saw a man who appeared to be dying of respiratory obstruction. When a worm wriggled from his windpipe and out his mouth, he promptly recovered.

Since these parasites can cause so much trouble, I tried, except in emergencies, to eliminate them before operating. More than ninety percent of the patients were infested with them and they were a constant source of anxiety.

Hookworms too were common. The presence of such permanent boarders has a bad effect on health and reduces the amount of nourishment available to the host from the food he eats.

The frequency of intestinal parasites is largely due to the unsanitary age-old habit of disposing nightsoil on fields without any treatment to destroy the parasite eggs. Not realizing the seriousness of parasite infestation and taking it as a matter of course, farmers didn't want to go to the trouble or expense of rendering such fertilizer safe and many were not aware that it could be done.

Another type of parasite—lung and liver flukes—for which

no satisfactory treatment was known, sapped the strength of numbers of people. The former was supposed to die out naturally after about fifteen years if the unfortunate host lived that long.

I was once summoned to the room of a colleague to see him remove what appeared to be a worm from the eye of a patient. Actually the parasite came from beneath the delicate covering of the eyeball, not from the interior of the eye. Neither of us had seen or read of such a parasite, or of one in such a location, but it wasn't long before the doctor found similar ones in different locations. While closing an abdominal incision after an operation, he discovered one in the abdominal wall. In another case, a man complained of a small painless but rapidly growing lump on his back. On examining the little cystlike mass, the surgeon observed motion inside it. He made a small incision and picked out a wormlike parasite two inches long.

Next to parasite infestations, the most frequent condition was stomach trouble of one kind or another. Probably the large amounts of red pepper in the Korean diet had something to do with that. Food that burns the lips is quite likely to have a similar effect on the lining of the stomach.

Dietetic treatment was ineffectual since no patient would follow a diet. He thought he might as well suffer from his disease as from starvation, and any diet that did not allow large quantities of rice and kimche containing red pepper was considered practically starvation. Patients wanted to be treated by large doses of powerful medicine, preferably injected. The amount of money and medicine that was, and still is, wasted on useless preparations supposed to promote digestion would have built some of the needed schools. Koreans are not alone in misuse of drugs.

The exit from the stomach was often so narrowed by scar tissue surrounding an old ulcer that it was almost completely obstructed. Some of these patients were literally starving, since the food eaten could not pass on from the stomach in anything like adequate quantities. Some patients came with a perforated ulcer and stomach contents leaking into the abdominal cavity, or with profuse hemorrhage requiring immediate surgery.

These patients were warned not to take solid food till the stomach wound had time to heal. After the first twenty-four hours, they were fed carefully with small amounts of fluids for some days. One morning, on making ward rounds, I was horrified to see a man who'd had an extensive stomach operation the previous afternoon sitting straight up in bed polishing off the bottom of a large bowl of macaroni, pork, and vegetables.

"Do you want to die?" I cried out.

"Not at all," he replied. "I've been starved for years and now I'm cured I'm going to enjoy eating again."

From then on, he had three square meals a day and a few extra things his friends brought him, and he did well. After that experience, I put a couple of extra stitches in the stomach wound where it would have the most strain and let the patients eat what they wanted. It didn't hurt them and they would almost certainly get it anyway since visiting friends often brought food, such as dried raw squid, a special delicacy much favored by visitors. I never saw any bad results from letting patients have solid food as soon as they wanted it after surgery. Years later, Western surgeons began giving their postoperative patients more food sooner than before, and with good results.

Eating before an operation was a different matter.

A twelve-year-old boy was brought to the hospital at night with acute appendicitis. Since the condition was of only short duration and the lighting uncertain, I decided to wait till morning before operating. The parents were warned not to let the child have anything to eat until told it would be safe to do so. Next morning, just to be sure, I asked them if he had eaten anything. On being assured he'd had nothing, I proceeded with the operation. As it was an uncomplicated case, the surgery was soon completed. While being transferred to a stretcher to be carried back to the ward, the child began to wake up. As he did so, he vomited a large amount of sticky half-chewed rice, aspirated some of it into his windpipe, and as he was still not conscious enough to cough it up, he died of suffocation right there in the operating room. The parents saw what had happened and realized too late that they themselves had caused the death of their son.

"Why did you give him all that rice?" I demanded. "Didn't I tell you not to give him anything before the operation?"

"Yes," said the mother, "but we didn't think it would matter, and we were afraid he'd be hungry." This was one case where the surgeon wasn't blamed for the death of the patient. Later, when we had a suction machine, a death of this sort could be prevented.

On making rounds another day, I found a man operated on the previous afternoon for a ruptured hernia missing from the ward. No one had seen him leave and we began to fear his family had spirited him off in the night. Just then, he came walking into the room.

"You gave us all a scare," I said reproachfully. "You don't need to go to the bathroom by yourself yet. The nurses and orderlies are here to bring you anything you need."

"I'd be ashamed to ask them to wait on me when I can look after myself," he replied.

In those days, surgical textbooks taught that hernia patients should be kept in bed for ten days in order to avoid strain on the wound until it had time to heal firmly. This was my first experience with what a few years later was hailed as a great advance in the postoperative care of surgical cases—including hernia—who were made to walk a few steps the day after the operation. In Korea, we discovered the advantages of early exercise and practiced it years before it became general policy in the West.

Maternity cases often were more worrisome than surgical ones. Normal ones seldom came to hospital. Husbands and mothers-in-law saw no reason to waste good money on unnecessary medical care. Hadn't babies been born for thousands of years without doctors or midwives?

I dreaded to see a maternity case come because so many were in such serious condition that mother or child or both were in danger and frequently the baby was already dead. Mothers seldom came until they had been two or more days in labor, completely exhausted, and often infected from unwise and unskilled attempts to deliver the baby. Because doctors were seldom called, they had little experience in the care of difficult labor. In cases that would have required a Cesarean section, when we first saw the mother, it was usually on account of an infection and, therefore, too late for that operation to be safely performed. This, of course, was before the days of antibiotics or sulfa drugs.

One who came early was a girl of seventeen brought by her sixty-year-old husband. Tuberculosis of the lower spine during childhood resulted in a large hump on her lower back. Both hip joints were completely fused with the thighs flexed on the body and the knees approximated. It was impossible for a child to be born naturally through the deformed and contracted pelvis.

Such a cripple couldn't expect much in the way of a husband. Neither could an old man of ordinary means expect a smart young woman as a wife, but since he had no son, he had to make the best bargain a go-between could manage. Probably each was disappointed on seeing the other at their wedding.

The deformed and crippled mother had been in labor for twenty-four hours and the baby appeared to be dead. An abdominal operation was necessary.

That had its problems too. The mother was bent almost double at the hips. She couldn't lie on her back on account of the hump. With her lying in a semilateral position, her chest bent forward, and her thighs flexed on her body, there wasn't much space in which to operate. Before undertaking the surgery, I tried to persuade the parents to agree to sterilization since further pregnancies, unless the woman could quickly get to a hospital, would be perilous. They wouldn't consent. The baby was dead, and they must try again to get a son to carry on the family name. It didn't matter about the mother. She could be replaced.

Not much more than a year later they returned, earlier this time. Another operation was performed and again they refused sterilization since the baby, though living, was only a girl. The subsequent history I never knew.

I had to deal with all the textbook complications and others as well.

While on furlough, I once asked a professor of obstetrics and gynecology what he would do when faced with a complicated case I described to him.

"I'd cut her throat," he replied, which council of despair wasn't very helpful.

One common complication of childbirth was narrowing of the birth canal from contraction of scar tissue following the burning treatments for descent of the uterus and bladder following neglected labor. As these unfortunates generally came to the hospital only after two or more days of trial labor at home and after unskilled attempts at delivery by a neighbor, they were usually already infected. An abdominal delivery in such cases was likely to result in fatal peritonitis. If the child were still alive on arrival, local surgery usually saved both mother and baby.

In order to encourage women to come for prenatal care, I set a regular charge for complete maternity care. This included five monthly prenatal examinations and a final checkup a month after the baby came. They could pay for each examination as they had it, the amount being deducted from the total cost of the delivery. Paying by such installments made it easier to pay the bill. Women felt they were getting something for nothing as the charge was the same whether or not they had the prenatal examinations. This induced a good many to come for prenatal examination and advice, which in turn, prevented some difficulties.

Delivering complicated maternity patients even in the hospital with facilities and assistance available could be troublesome enough. But with the patient on the floor in a tiny ill-lighted room without an assistant, it is doubly difficult. When called to such patients in their homes, I used to urge the family to bring the woman to the hospital where we could do more for her. They usually said she was too sick to come which was often true since the journey often involved jolting for two or more hours in a springless bull cart. Even though I couldn't do all in a home that could be done in the hospital, on considering the alternative—mistreatment or mutilation at the hands of some ignorant old woman—I went and did my best.

On one such occasion, I found the baby in a transverse position. An arm had been delivered and the doctor, who had been called at this stage, cut it off just below the shoulder, and took his departure. The child was dead and the mother in a serious condition. Sprawling around on the floor, it was impossible to keep my apron sterile. I did the best I could under the circumstances. With difficulty, I succeeded in changing the position and delivering the baby. The mother made a good recovery.

One cold winter night I was getting ready for bed after late rounds in the hospital when Kang Do-Ka knocked on the door. She told me four men from a village on the plain across the river had come to take me to see a woman in difficult labor. It wasn't far, they said, no more than ten *li*—about three miles. They'd brought a rickshaw puller with his vehicle. "But it's very late," Do-Ka said, "and cold and snowing. Don't go tonight. Wait till morning."

I thought she was being over solicitous on my behalf. Having long since decided I'd never let a call go unheeded if it were physically possible to get there, I wrapped up warmly and we set out. The snow was only an inch or two deep and, guided by the men, we made good time to the village which proved to be fifteen *li* distant.

The whole village seemed to be gathered in the yard, not wholly out of concern for the patient, I suspected, but to have a look at the foreign doctor as well.

Five or six women were in the seven-foot-square room

with the distressed mother. Some were holding her hands, others giving advice, and the biggest one there was pressing with her feet on the patient's back as the mother crouched, hands and knees on the floor. A wick burning in a saucer of oil on a brass stand gave the only light. At my request for more light, they brought a candle.

I asked three of the onlookers to step outside to give me room to work. With obvious reluctance, they did. Then I got a small, low table and proceeded to set out sterile supplies. The dear old grandmother, eager to help, smoothed out the sterile towel covering the table with hands none too clean. Begging her to desist did no good at all. She was determined to be useful. Flies found in hot floor rooms all winter long kept alighting on the sterile goods.

Fortunately, during the long hours the mother had been in labor, she'd made considerable progress and didn't require much help. The baby after its ordeal had to be resuscitated.

As soon as it was born, the mother anxiously asked, "What is it? What is it?"

"Only a girl," replied the women in disgusted chorus.

"A useless thing has been born," said the disappointed mother. "The baby's father will be very sorry."

That attitude used to distress me, but after the initial disappointment was past, usually the little girls were loved and well cared for, though not pampered the way boys were.

The grandmother helpfully fetched a dirty kitchen knife to cut the cord. I'm afraid she felt her assistance wasn't appreciated when I used my sterile scissors instead.

Then she brought a large bowl of seaweed soup, given to all mothers of newborn babies, and insisted on the weary woman sitting up and drinking it at once.

"Why make her drink it now?" I asked. "She's exhausted after all those hours of pain and effort. Let her rest a while first."

They all looked at me. Foreign doctors evidently didn't know much since it was common knowledge that a new mother had to have seaweed soup the minute the baby was born or she'd never be able to nurse it and the child would starve.

While the mother drank the soup, the infant was passed around from one to another of the nursing mothers present and several more had come in. Each of them gave it her breast.

In preparation for the birth, the straw matting had been removed from the floor and replaced by loose straw. One woman now took some of this, wrapped the placenta in it, and stood the bundle up in one corner of the room to remain there until the baby's cord dropped off.

Village women helping on such occasions sometimes used a sharp blade of coarse grass to saw through the cord that was left several inches long. Due to such methods, numbers of babies died of tetanus within a few days of birth. How so many manage to survive is a mystery probably understood only in Heaven. Before the birth, the mother had donned her dirtiest clothes since they would have to be washed anyway. As no one knew whether it would live or not, nothing had been provided for the baby. A moderately clean towel and a bit of dirty blanket were produced for the child. After making the mother clean and comfortable, I placed the baby on the hot floor beside her, and set out for home about three o'clock in the morning. The crowd had dispersed and all the village lights were out. New snow had fallen on the narrow paths and covered our tracks. There were no guides on the homeward way, but the father of the unwelcome daughter pointed out the direction of the city fifteen *li* distant, and we started.

The snow ceased to fall, the sky was clear, and the rickshaw man, after walking for half an hour, thought we should be able to make out the city lights. After plodding on for another half hour and still not being able to make out the lights, he woke the people in a house we were passing and asked how far it was to Hamheung.

"Fifteen *li*," was the reply.

"What direction is it from here?" The main pointed, and we set off again.

We were both tired and sleepy when to our surprise we found ourselves back in the village where our patient lived. There was still a light in that house, and they had a great laugh at us when we asked the way to Hamheung. Once more we started for the city, still fifteen *li* distant.

Paths wove among the rice fields, but there was no road on that part of the plain and, on account of the newly fallen snow, not a track but our own could be seen.

The night was getting colder. We were both weary and I was sorry for the poor fellow who had to pull a rickshaw with me aboard so far through the snow. We decided to stop somewhere nearby and rest till daylight.

At the next village we stopped at the gate of a house where several stacks of grain in the yard indicated an affluent household. Here there might be space for traveling strangers lost on the plain. Shouts at the gate brought out the dogs. The rickshaw man continued calling and finally a man appeared. We explained our predicament and asked if we might stay till daylight when we could find our way. I got out of the vehicle to let the man see I was a woman and take me to the women's quarters. He told us to go around the nearest corner of the house and enter the first door we came to.

We stepped into a room about seven feet square where four men were sleeping. Waking up, they asked who we were and the cause of the interruption this time of night. The rickshaw man explained. I was still hoping someone would come to take me to the women's part of the house, but no one did and the man who had admitted us had disappeared. I couldn't go wandering about a strange house in the dark.

One of the occupants of the room lighted the wick in the saucer of oil on a low stand. The only other item of furnishing the room could boast was a large brass chamber pot which they invited me to use. Under the circumstances, I declined. They handed me one of the wooden blocks they were using for pillows. As there wasn't room for six to stretch out on the floor, I settled in for the hours till daylight by half leaning up against the wall in one corner. It was so cold I was glad to keep my coat on, and the rickshaw man had the blanket out of his two-wheeler. Presently, finding my position uncomfortable, I tried cautiously to change it a little without disturbing others.

"Here, you nearest the lamp," said a voice, "light the wick. She's trying to find the chamber pot."

I didn't move again no matter how cramped my position was. Whatever would my mother say if she could see me now, I thought as I dozed off.

As the first streak of dawn filtered through the paper window, we were up and away without awaking anyone. In a short time, we saw the smoke arising from the morning fires in the city, and as we crossed the long bridge over the river, the sun rose over Dragon Hill.

-11-

In two years, the work increased so that I could not carry it alone. A call to the country left the hospital with no doctor till my return. When the mission station decided to engage another doctor to share the work and make expansion possible, a fellow missionary in another hospital recommended Dr. Hong, a capable man in internal medicine. He took over the medical work while I had surgery, administration, and obstetrics and gynecology. We now had consultations in difficult cases. Dr. Hong assisted in major surgery and one of us took country or house calls while the other carried on in the hospital.

Viola Cardwell finished her studies at language school and now began regular instructions for the nursing attendants. Under her teaching and supervision, they soon became more efficient.

Viola brought her language teacher, Chang Sunsaing, from Seoul as her assistant and matron of the nurses' dormitory. She also had responsibility for the food served to nurses and patients. The two made a fine team. The wards became cleaner and neater, the food better, and the nursing service greatly improved.

The nurses had been living in two old thatched mud

houses where the cooking for both nurses and patients was done over fires on the level of the kitchen floor. We needed something better. Our mission board provided funds to which replace these dilapidated buildings with a brick dormitory on the hill behind the hospital. The new building also contained a kitchen for the hospital.

Now we were making progress and thought we should do something to provide medical care farther afield. In the town of Hongwon, two hours north by train from Hamheung, there was no medical doctor for a population of about ten thousand. We decided to open a clinic there. After arranging with the local church people to give some assistance, we rented, repaired, and improved an old Korean house making it more suitable for our work. The clinic was to be open one day weekly.

As the building could not be left unoccupied all week, we sent Yum Nu-Ka, who had married and changed his name from Nu-Ka to Ke-Moon, to live in the house in Hongwon. He was much more than a caretaker. He was nurse, dispenser, and general factotum in the new clinic. He and his wife lived in one of the rooms of the three-room house.

Taking medicines and supplies with us each time, Dr. Hong and I took turns going to the weekly clinic. There was a walk of a mile to the station in Hamheung and the same distance to the clinic in Hongwon. Trains were never clean and in the winter never warm. Spitting and throwing trash on the floor was a matter of course. What cleaning was done consisted of flooding the floor with water to keep down dust and then, with a short-handled broom, sweeping empty cardboard boxes, cigarette stubbs, bits of paper, apple peelings, eggshells, broken chopsticks, and such clutter into the aisle and toward the door. Anything hard to reach was left behind. In winter, the water froze on the floors and, except in the immediate vicinity of the smoky coal stove in the middle of the car, never thawed. The men passengers congregated around the stove, but sometimes I squeezed in long enough to warm my feet that quickly grew cold again on the icy floor.

Yum would be at the station to carry the bags. It was good to get out into the fresh air after the smoke and fumes of the grimy train, and I was glad to walk fast to get warmed up.

Patients came with all sorts of complaints. I urged seriously ill people and those requiring surgery to go to the Cheihei Hospital. Frequently they did, often considerably later and after spending their little money at the native practitioner's on such remedies as deerhorn, concoctions of snakes and lizards, and other equally effective remedies.

At our clinic, most people wanted a large syringeful of colored liquid shot directly into the blood. This they considered more efficacious than medicine taken by mouth. Some who refused ordinary medicine were willing to pay for injections.

Few had watches or clocks, but Yum explained how to take their medicine.

"When the train whistle blows in the morning," he told them, "take the first dose. When the sun's right overhead in the middle of the day take another spoonful, and when the night train blows take the third dose. *Don't* take it all at once."

"How many days will it take to cure me?"

"You should soon begin to feel better. If you aren't a lot better in a few days come back next week and let the doctor see you again."

I spent as much time as possible teaching about sanitation and good health habits in the hope that at least some would adopt new ideas and try to follow them.

Fairly often, while I was in Hŏngwon, some emergency surgical case would come to the Cheihei Hospital, and finding no surgeon there, would leave, or wait till I got back at seven in the evening. Seriously ill patients in Hongwon needed to be seen more often than once a week, but with the clinic open only one day in seven, the income wasn't sufficient to pay expenses. So, when a qualified doctor began practice in the town a year or two later, we closed the dispensary, which was no longer needed, and devoted full time to the hospital.

Hospital problems were not the only ones.

On returning from annual mission meeting at Wonsan Beach, I found a delegation from Yungsaing Girls' School staff waiting for me. When one of the pupils failed to return to school after the summer holiday, they had investigated the reason. Her mother had died some years before and when her father recently died an uncle became her guardian. Seeing no reason to support his niece—let alone educate her—he sold the girl.

"For gracious sakes!" I exclaimed in surprised distress. "Is that possible in this country?"

"Yes, Japanese law permits it, and her guardian has authority to do as he pleases. She's only a girl and is now the property of the man who bought her. She can't help herself."

"That's dreadful! Isn't there some way she can escape such a fate?"

"Only if we buy her back. We've taken up a collection in the school for that purpose, but we haven't enough and we've come to ask you to help."

"How much more do you need?"

"Fifty yen." Twenty-five dollars.

"I'll give that," I said.

"We've raised a hundred at the school. Here it is. Take it and please go right away and buy her," pleaded the teacher. "We shouldn't wait any longer or she might be sent away."

"Why don't you buy her?" I asked, appalled at the idea of my buying another human being. "What kind of rumors might circulate if a missionary were known to buy a girl?"

"We can't possibly buy her," replied the teacher. "The school can't buy her. If it got about that a man teacher, or a school in which there are men teachers, bought one of the pupils, there would be such a scandal the school would be ruined. Parents would take their daughters out of the school. *You* must buy her. Everybody knows that if a woman missionary bought a girl, it would be to save her from the fate for which girls are usually bought."

"How old is she, and what's her name? Who owns her and

where can we find him? Someone must come with me on business like this."

"One of the women teachers and the chaplain will go with you. You're right. It wouldn't do to try to handle this alone. She's sixteen and her name's Ko Soon-Hi. Her owner keeps a brothel in Kumi Dong. You can't buy a girl like a piece of furniture. She's more like real estate and you have to go to the police station and have the transaction registered there. We'll get in touch with the man who bought her and arrange for him to meet you at the police station at the end of the bridge at one o'clock today. The chaplain and Song Sunsaing will come and take you there."

"Shouldn't the girl come too?"

"The man will have to bring her to hand her over to you after the purchase."

"What if he refuses?"

"He won't. It would hurt his reputation to have his name in the papers over such an affair—buying a girl right after her father's death like that. We'll tell him we'll give the whole story to the papers if he doesn't agree to let us buy her back."

Song Sunsaing explained the matter to the police. The brothel keeper wanted to make a good profit on the deal. The Japanese policeman said it was very generous of the school and the missionary to set the girl free and he must sell her for the same price he paid.

I handed over the hundred and fifty yen and received a receipt. The sympathetic policeman made out papers stating that the girl was now my property and could not be claimed by either the uncle or the brothel keeper.

What was I to do next? After her experience, she couldn't go back to school or the other pupils would leave. One of the women teachers took her home with her for a few days while arrangements were being made with the Salvation Army in Seoul. They took her into their Girls' Home and taught her sewing and dressmaking and later she was married from there.

Only once more did I ever buy anybody.

Our hospital woman evangelist, Cho Rachel, told me a sad story she heard from a young woman in a house where she was preaching. Following a long illness, the woman's husband had died in the government hospital in the northern city of Hoiryung. The hospital demanded the wife pay the bill. She'd already paid as much as she could from the sale of all her possessions, but the hospital insisted she must pay more. To get the money, she sold herself for a period of ten years, by which time she would have worked off the purchase price and be free.

After several years in a Japanese brothel in that town, she was transferred to one in Hamheung. She was so sick of that kind of life she would have done anything to get away. She appealed to the police for help, but they told her she must stick to the bargain and, if they heard of her trying to run away, they'd see she was not only sent back, but punished as well.

"What kind of person does she seem to be?" I asked.

"She's never been to school, but she's clean and gentle and looks sad. She didn't seem a bad type at all. I believe what she said about being sick of the life she has to live."

"How much more time has she to put in?"

"Another year and a half and she says she can't stand it that long. She might take poison."

"That means a good deal of her debt has been worked off. It shouldn't cost too much to buy her out now. How much do you think?"

"I don't know, but I'll find out," said Rachel, starting for the door.

"Go and have another talk with her. See if she has any relatives she could go to and if there's anything else she can do to make a living. Find out exactly how much she still owes."

Rachel hurried away, to return in an hour with the woman who was overjoyed at the hope of becoming free without finishing out her servitude. The sum needed was fifty yen.

Rachel went with me and I paid the money as before.

When she received the paper giving her her freedom she prostrated herself before me in gratitude. She too went to the Salvation Army Home where she learned to read and write and found a better way to make a living. Several times she wrote to thank me and tell me how happy she was in her new life. Then a letter came saying she had found joy and peace of mind in the knowledge that she was forgiven and Jesus was her Savior and friend. Within a year or two, she was married and once more had the security of a home of her own.

Such were not the only experiences outside medical work.

A gentle knock on my door one night announced the presence of Kang Do-Ka.

"Pouine," said she, "Are you warm, comfortable, at peace?" No one else called me that, but it was Do-Ka's name for me. Everyone else called me *Wonjang, Won* for hospital, *jang* meaning straight—literally, the one who keeps the hospital straight, otherwise superintendent or administrator. The name Murray was difficult for a Korean tongue to pronounce and became Mori. Hence I was known as Mori Wonjang. *Pouine* was Do-Ka's name for Dr. MacMillan and she transferred the name along with her allegiance to me.

"Pouine," said she, "on Saturday afternoon I'm going to a village where a *mudang* and her family have become Christians. They want me to destroy the devil things in their house. Come with me. Have you ever seen the devil things in a Korean house?"

"No, I haven't, and I'll certainly go unless some emergency case comes to keep me in the hospital. But, if they've become Christians, why do they need you to destroy the fetishes? Can't they do it themselves?"

"They want them destroyed. They believe in God, but the mother's been a *mudang* and they've feared evil spirits for so long they can't quite get up courage enough to do it themselves."

On Saturday afternoon we walked about four miles to the village on the great rice plain across the river. The former *mudang* met us at the entrance to the village where stood two fierce looking figures carved from wooden posts. Chinese characters written on them proclaimed that one was the greatest general under Heaven, the other his wife. Many villages were still guarded by such "devil posts." Escorted by the former *mudang*, we entered her courtyard where the rest of the family was waiting. After the customary greetings and low bows all around, the woman thanked us for coming and said how ashamed she was at having all these devil things in her house and how happy she would be to get rid of them.

"Where are the devil things?" asked Kang Do-Ka. "Let's get to work on them."

The son of the household had been to school and lost faith in the powers of the spirits some time before, but his mother refused to let him touch the fetishes. He now led the way to a small dark room at the back of the house set aside for the spirits. The tiny room was filled with dusty worn-out baskets and rusty old pails containing handfuls of different grains offered to the spirits from the first fruits of each harvest. There were cracked clay pots with bits of feathers from fowls sold or eaten at feasts, pieces of material from each garment made in the house over the years, and various other cast-off odds and ends.

Kang Do-Ka emptied these things out to the accompaniment of clouds of dust and piled them in a heap in the middle of the courtyard.

"Is that all?" demanded Do-Ka.

"No, Grandmother, not quite all," and they added more to the pile from another room.

"Are you sure there's no more?"

"Only these," said the converted sorceress bringing out a tattered and very dirty black gauze gown with red facings around the neck and down the front and a pair of brass cymbals.

"I wore this gown when exorcising spirits," she told us, "and these cymbals are charms that influenced them to leave." She handed the articles to Do-Ka who passed them over to me.

"Mori Pouine'll take these to Canada when she goes to

show people that this family is done with such futile things and now worships God."

The old baskets were added to the pile, the clay pots broken and flung in a heap in a corner of the yard together with the flattened old pails, so none of them could ever be used again. Then the pile in the yard was set on fire.

As flames consumed the devil things, the family, led by Do-Ka, sang hymns of triumph. When all were burnt up, they joined in a prayer of gratitude that the devils were gone and God had taken their place in their home and lives.

From then on, instead of charging exorbitantly to exorcise spirits she'd claimed were causing sickness, the former *mudang* advised the sick to go to the Christian hospital.

People who didn't believe that ordinary illnesses were caused by evil spirits were convinced that mental sickness was. Many firmly believed in devil possession. They didn't always call the sorceress, but sometimes took matters into their own hands. I've had patients brought to me after being severely beaten by their family in an attempt to drive out the spirits they thought were residing in the sick one. Such beatings were often repeated until the victim was badly injured, but I never knew of anyone's being improved by such cruel treatment.

Even some Christians believed in devil possession and tried methods of cure said to be successful in some cases. At a village church in the country, our hospital evangelist, Elder Lee, and I were asked to visit the home of a woman believed to be possessed. From what I heard and saw, I thought she was suffering from a fairly common form of mental illness.

The church people begged Elder Lee to drive out the evil spirit and he agreed to try. He read a portion of scripture, then all joined in singing hymns. The elder urged the woman to sing too, but she ignored him and was noisy and restless. Others prayed in turn, asking for release of the woman from the power of the spirit. The elder tried to persuade her to pray. She didn't, but during the prayers she became quiet and still. After the prayers, Elder Lee, in a loud voice, and in the least respectful language possible, ordered the spirit to come out.

"Wicked and hateful spirit," he shouted, leaning toward the woman. "Come out of this person. Come out at once, I say. Come out, and never trouble her again." The poor woman began to cry quietly and the tossing and flinging about ceased. I observed no other change and we had to leave then.

Later, we learned that nothing dramatic had taken place, but from the time we were there, the unfortunate woman gradually improved and was now almost well.

Nothing could be farther removed from that tormented woman than stolid Kim Wha-Soon, the middle-aged church worker from the little church across the river. After she had been there a couple of years, she came to our house one day to see Edna McLellan, friend and counselor of the women evangelists. After the proper polite greetings and inquiries, Wha-Soon hung her head and shyly broached the subject she had come to discuss.

"What would you think—" she hesitated. "What would you think of my getting married?"

Edna had supposed Wha-Soon was a widow or deserted wife and she was far past the time when a Korean woman was likely to get married.

"I thought you were married long ago," said Edna. "What happened? Did your husband die?"

Wha-Soon looked at the floor. "I don't know whether I was married or not," she said.

"What!" exclaimed Edna. "You don't know whether you were married or not! What do you mean?"

"Well, it was like this. When I was a small child my father had a very close friend who lived in the next village and he had a little son about my age. The two men thought it would be a happy thing if the families were united by marriage. They exchanged the customary engagement gifts, signed betrothal papers, and we two children at the ages of three and four were engaged to be married."

"But that wasn't marriage, only an engagement."

"Yes, but you know in our country the exchange of gifts and the signing of the papers is the legally binding thing, and the wedding ceremony just the announcement to the public. Anyway, when I was ten and the boy nine, they had the wedding feast, and the bridegroom and his parents spent the customary three days at our house, but we children were too shy to speak to one another or to be alone together. All agreed I was too young to leave my home, and the groom's party returned to their village while I remained with my parents. I never saw that boy again for he died the next year. Now, was I married, or wasn't I? Anyway I've been faithful to his memory for more than thirty years and that's a long time to live alone. I'm getting on, and beginning to think of what's going to happen to me in my old age. How'm I going to live?"

Drawing up her feet, she sat comfortably cross-legged in the big chair, her eyes still downcast.

"Are you thinking of anyone in particular?" asked Edna.

"Well," she paused shyly, "You know Kim Changno of Samsoo? A go-between has come from him to arrange a marriage if I agree. They say he was good to his first wife. She died six months ago, and he never had a son. His daughters are married and away, leaving no one to cook his rice and care for his old blind mother. He'd like a son too, of course, as he also has to think of his old age. If I agree to marry him, do you think I'd have a son? If not, I doubt if it'd be worthwhile." Wha-Soon looked anxiously at Edna.

"Why don't you ask Dr. Murray? She knows more about such things than I do."

"That's a good idea. Thank you for suggesting it. I'll go right now." She bustled off.

Ten minutes later Do-Ka's gentle *"Pouine,"* at my clinic door, announced her presence. "The evangelist from the church across the river is here to see you."

"Bring her in as soon as this patient leaves. It'll be only a few minutes. Is she sick?"

"She doesn't look sick. She wants to see you about something."

In a few minutes Wha-Soon's broad face and toothy grin appeared followed closely by Wha-Soon herself. "Are you in peace?"

"Yes. Are you? Is anything wrong?"

"Miss McLellan sent me to see you." She paused. The voluble Wha-Soon didn't often pause. Something must be wrong.

"What is it?" I asked.

"Kim Changno of Samsoo has sent a go-between—" The story came out.

"I see. No one can guarantee anybody's having a child, still less promise a son. How old are you?"

"Forty-three, and the elder's sixty, but we're both healthy and he's had several children, but only daughters."

"Stranger things have happened. It's worth taking a chance if you want to try it, but don't blame me or feel too disappointed if you don't get the son you'd like. Think it over well and pray about it before making up your mind."

Great was the excitement in the little church across the river. At the age of forty-three, their evangelist was going to be married. Whoever heard of such a thing with no relative to make a match for her and no one to give her a wedding feast. No wonder she'd been a long time getting married, they thought. Now that it was about to happen, they rose to the occasion. The church would give the feast and she would be married there.

The day came. The church was packed. When no more could get in at the door, some came in the windows, and those who couldn't stuck their heads in.

The elder looked proud and happy. His friends were there to congratulate him. It wasn't every widower of sixty who got a wife young enough to give him a son.

Wha-Soon, in a beautiful white silk wedding gown, looked as demure as a Korean bride should; never once did she raise her eyes. Not even the shadow of a smile crossed her face. But old customs, for Christians, at least, were becoming less rigid and she replied shyly to the good wishes of her friends the church people.

The feast did credit to those who prepared it and to the couple themselves. Everybody saw them off at the railway station and reports came later from the northern mountain village that the new daughter-in-law was as obedient to her husband and her mother-in-law as any wife should be and was pointed to as an example for all the young wives in the village.

-12-

It was a great day when we replaced the inadequate old sterilizer with a new and larger autoclave and secured enough laboratory equipment to do basic tests. We engaged a well-trained laboratory technician from another mission hospital and began better laboratory work.

I set a goal of one major advance every six months. It took so long to get the staff interested enough to make a change in methods or to try something new that it didn't seem possible to progress faster than that. For months before trying to start some new development, I mentioned to various members of the staff that they were trying something new in another hospital and wondered when we would be able to do it. After thus cultivating the ground, I called a staff meeting. If one of them suggested trying the new method or plan, it was as good as done. If I had to suggest it myself the response would be that such a plan might work all right in Canada, but not in Korea. If that was the attitude, the time wasn't ripe for the change, and it was wiser to wait till the staff were ready to cooperate.

One advance was the setting aside of a separate room for a maternity ward, apart from other patients some of whom would be suffering from infectious conditions. It took a long time to convince the staff of the desirability of this innovation. They were sure the mothers would be lonely, perhaps afraid, in a room by themselves, and wouldn't be willing to stay there.

It proved otherwise. Mothers were pleased to have a special room, and since we had no delivery room, normal cases, when there were such, were delivered in the maternity ward. The mothers preferred this to the operating room that was used for complicated cases.

The next advance was converting the sitting room Miss Hall and I had shared into a children's ward. This was in the wing over the outpatient clinic away from the general wards, so that the small patients would disturb others as little as possible.

With cribs nicely painted in cheerful colors, gay quilts sent by women's groups in Canada, and little bedside tables, the room looked quite attractive. An exception was a number of long benches that all assured me we *must* provide for the home attendants, without whom no family would think of allowing a child to be admitted. Mother or grandmother couldn't be expected to sleep on the cold floor. Unless she had a bench, she would curl up in the crib with the child and both would be uncomfortable.

Some of my planned advances were not achieved.

I hoped the time had come when we could organize a hospital auxiliary to make sheets, pillowcases, and pajamas and do mending for the hospital. This would save the salary of a sewing woman and leave more money for free treatment for the poor. Equally important, I hoped it would encourage the group to do something for those outside their own families.

Korean culture provided that anyone in need was cared for by some member of the family even if not very closely related. Anyone else was some other family's responsibility and others were not concerned. Orphanages were hardly needed, and few existed in those days since orphans were looked after as a matter of course by the family group. The few without families fared badly in sickness or old age.

Older women had daughters-in-law to do the work and I hoped they might be willing to give one or two afternoons a month to sewing for the hospital. Worn sheets and pajamas needed mending and replacement.

When I suggested this to Chang Sunsaing, the hospital matron, she was aghast.

"That'll be too expensive for the hospital," she objected.

"Expensive!" I said. "It's to save expense I'm suggesting it. Surely a group of Christian women would be glad to give a little time to help the hospital to care for poor patients."

"We'd have to buy all new materials for them to work on and that will cost money. We couldn't possibly ask them to mend pajamas or sheets that had been used."

"Why not? They'd be clean and fresh from the laundry."

"Impossible," declared Chang Sunsaing firmly.

"Well, we need some new sheets, don't we? Let's buy a couple of bolts of unbleached cotton and begin with that."

"But we've only one sewing machine. We need one for each woman who comes."

"Do they all have sewing machines at home? And they all sew, don't they?"

"Not many of them have sewing machines, but *we* couldn't ask them to come and sew for the hospital without giving them a machine to use."

"What's the difference between sewing by hand at home and doing it here? Besides, if they make pajamas, some could cut out and some sew on buttons."

"We'll have to give them a big dinner and that will cost more than the value of the work they'll do."

"Why will we have to give them a big dinner? If they work from two till four in the afternoon wouldn't a cup of tea and a cookie be enough?"

"That's not Korean custom."

"Let's try to find a way to get people to do something to help others. I'm going to talk about this at the next meeting of the women's evangelistic society in the church across the river and see what they think."

"That might be all right in Canada, but it won't work in Korea."

When I spoke to the women about it in the church group, they were enthusiastic. Of course they'd go, but not for just two hours. That would hardly be worthwhile. They would go in the morning and work all day.

I told them we would be grateful for two hours and couldn't think of having them work all day.

"That's fine," they said. "We'll be there bright and early day after tomorrow."

When she heard this, Chang Sunsaing was flabbergasted.

She went to the market and bought straw matting to spread on the floor of the room where the women would sew. She bought two bolts of cotton goods for them to make into sheets. I had to borrow two sewing machines from rather unwilling missionaries who weren't exactly enthusiastic over the idea of learners practicing on their machines.

On the appointed day, a dozen women arrived at nine o'clock. Someone had to be with them to show them what to do and how to do it.

Since they came for the day, they had to have lunch which Chang Sunsaing ordered from a restaurant downtown. It was delivered in bowls together with a kettle of soy sauce and another of soup balanced on a twelve-foot-long plank by a boy riding a bicycle. Not a drop was spilled.

The auxiliary worked well, but a sewing woman could have done the work in three days for less than it cost the hospital to provide for and feed the voluntary helpers. I charged the expense up to experience, and the auxiliary ceased to function.

Some of the advances adopted still left us with problems.

There was no danger of children falling out of cribs if the sides were left up, but the mothers generally took at least one side down and half sat in the crib themselves. If a younger child died, the mother often resumed nursing the next older, so the milk wouldn't be wasted, and some children were nursed till four or even five years old. I knew one boy who used to run home from school at noon time to be nursed.

Often several family members wanted to stay with the small patient to care for him and see his progress for themselves. We tried to limit the number to one since there just wasn't room enough in the six-crib ward for the doctors and nurses to do their work with eight or ten adults standing around in the way.

As the hospital couldn't afford to feed mothers and visitors free, and they couldn't afford to have food sent in from an inn or restaurant, they often shared the patient's food. The sick one thus was deprived of needed nourishment by the very people insisting on caring for him.

When a mother wanted to sleep, she often changed off with the grandmother who couldn't be taught anything. Grandmothers, having had seven or eight children of their own, thought they knew all there was to know about babies and children and how to look after them. That half of theirs had died in infancy was quite irrelevant to them. They liked to carry not only small babies, but quite large children up and down the corridors and into other patients' rooms on their backs.

When a child was very sick, I used to plead with the grandmother to let him lie quietly in his crib, but she seldom paid any attention. Once, when I remonstrated with an old woman for carrying her grandchild on her back only an hour after the child had had abdominal surgery, she said *"Yei, Yei"* ("Yes, Yes"), but made no move to do as I asked.

"Do put the baby in his crib," I urged. "Carrying him like that hurts him and hinders healing. Don't you want him to get well as soon as possible? Please put him down in his crib."

"Yei, Yei."

Next time I went to the children's ward the child might, in a sense, be said to be in the crib. The old lady was standing up in it, grandson still tied to her back. I gave up. Grandmothers were among the biggest problems in the hospital.

Sometimes I found a sick child on the floor under a crib, the mother sleeping in it, her legs hanging uncomfortably over the end. Waking the mother, I told her the crib was for the sick child and to put him back in it. She said the baby was used to the floor, but she'd never slept in a bed and wanted to see what it was like. What was unreasonable about that?

I've thanked the Lord for giving me a sense of humor, for I was often so exasperated, that if I couldn't laugh, I would have cried.

On various occasions, relatives, thinking a cast on a fractured limb was hurting the patient, removed the cast. It didn't occur to them that it was the injury that caused the pain. After this interference, if the family permitted, I reapplied the cast, sometimes having first to reduce the fracture over again. In case the family refused to have anything done and took the patient to another doctor, any bad result was likely to be blamed on our treatment. There was nothing to laugh about in such cases.

Bedpans were another problem. These were kept on a rack in the utility room where none but staff were allowed to enter. Such rules didn't deter family attendants. They went and got a bedpan when one was wanted, and after use, emptied it near the front gate, threw the contents from the nearest window, set it in the corridor as it was, or shoved it under the bed for use again. Night nurses, too, regularly distributed bedpans under beds at night to save themselves the trouble of getting them when wanted.

Family attendants thought the hospital a fine place to get the household washing done with hospital hot water and soap —luxuries few had at home. On late rounds or emergency calls at night, I frequently found a home attendant or other visitor in the utility room doing the family wash in the hopper. People accustomed to doing laundry in the river didn't realize that heating water cost money or that hot water wasn't quite as abundant as river water. During the washing, they left both tap and drain pipe fully open, the water running away full blast. When the drain got stopped up, as it frequently did, one often found in it a sock or small garment from somebody's wash.

Clothing drying on the radiators, stair rails, or front fence, though hardly attractive to look at, was not as serious as the loss of hot water needed for hospital purposes.

Patients and attendants alike insisted on windows being tightly closed. A ward for eight people gets very stuffy when there are a dozen visitors and all windows closed. On admitting a patient, the admitting officer explained that the hospital provided nursing care and family attendants were unnecessary. However, if the family insisted, one person was allowed to stay, but others often sneaked back into the wards after late rounds from where they had been hiding in the bathroom or behind a door.

It wasn't always possible to send visitors away at night. In the long summer days, farmers worked in the fields till dark, then had supper, and after that, would walk to the hospital to see a friend. Often they arrived after ten at night when lights were out and patients asleep. They frequently came in a group bringing food. Nothing else would do. They must see their friend and make sure he got the food by watching him eat it. It didn't matter to them that he was sleeping soundly and had to be awakened. It was useless to ask them not to disturb the whole ward or to leave the food and return in visiting hours the next day. Having come to see their friend, they intended to see him even if everybody in the hospital was disturbed. People could go to sleep again, couldn't they?

One visitor who used to come at night was the mother of a seven-year-old boy suffering from chronic bone infection. The mentally disturbed father beat his wife so cruelly she had to leave him. Since he came and went as he liked during the day, the mother visited her child at night. For coolness in the summer heat, the boy's crib was on the veranda.

One night, after the mother arrived, the father unexpectedly returned. The night nurse saw him coming and warned the mother who had time only to slip under the crib on to the concrete floor. Here she remained in a cramped position in constant fear of her husband's detecting her or the child inadvertently betraying her presence. Fortunately, it was dark on the veranda. The nurse hovered around in dread of what might happen. On her rounds, Kang Do-Ka grasped the situation and came for me.

"Do come and send the man away before he notices his wife and beats her up," she said. I went.

"I know you like to be with your boy," I told him, "but you've had a good visit now, and it's time for him to go to sleep. Come back in the morning."

"I don't want to go."

"Sleep is good for Hong-Siki. Don't you want him to get well soon? He can't sleep while you're talking to him."

"I didn't come to talk," said the father. "I came to bring him some candy."

"All right. Give him the candy and come back in the morning."

At last he got up to go; I accompanied him out the gate lest he should change his mind and return. He started to go back more than once, but I finally saw him turn the corner and disappear in the darkness. On being assured that he was gone, the mother emerged from under the crib, rubbed her stiff knees, and stole off in another direction.

Not all visitors came at inconvenient times.

One bright morning, when the clouds rode high in the sky and the rice fields on the plain were at their deepest emerald, Kim Wha-Soon, the former evangelist from the church across the river, arrived off the night train. After greeting us all in the hospital, she went off to see old friends in the church where she had been married.

That evening she was admitted as a patient and the elder had his long-hoped-for son. Wha-Soon was a proud woman. The elder's friends congratulated him, no longer addressed him as Elder Kim but Father of the Son. Everyone was happy over the good fortune of the little family, who, three days later, left for their home in a northern village, a day's journey by bull cart from their nearest railway station.

Hospitals in Korea may be affected very much by the

weather. Every rainy season, usually beginning early in July and lasting about a month, brings floods to some part of the country. One year it rained continually in our district for days, till the ground could absorb no more. Irrigation canals and rivers were overflowing their banks. Beside the city, the generally placid Sungchun River rose out of its channel and covered the wide area of sand between the embankments on each side. Still it rained, and still the river rose, till it was perilously near the top of the dikes. Through the years, the riverbed had filled with silt and sand till it was higher than some of the city streets in the lower part of the town.

While the flood lasted, the dikes were patroled day and night, and any places where the water began to erode, the banks were strengthened with bags of sand. But still the water rose—now a raging torrent. From Dragon Hill, the roaring of the waters sounded like ocean surf in a storm beating on a rocky coast with a thunderous terrifying sound.

I saw floating on the river bodies of drowned farm animals, roofs of houses, sheds, gates, logs, bridges, and small islands green with turf, torn from the riverbanks by the raging waters. As I watched, a long section of a bridge came rushing downstream toward the Mansei Bridge linking the city with the rice plain beyond and crashed into the Mansei Bridge. Both were swept down the river together and carried out to sea.

Though the dikes held, water began to overflow and soon backed up into the lower part of the city, thus causing great damage. A mud house can't stand much water before the flues beneath the floor, built of flat stones plastered together with clay, begin to collapse as the clay is washed away. Deeper water melts away the lower parts of the walls and the upper part, left without support, goes too. Next, the wooden frame falls, and doors, window frames, and corner posts float away, with them the contents of the house.

This flood not only did serious damage in the lower part of the city, but also to stock, crops, roads, and farmland in the upper reaches of the river. In places, the very soil was washed away. This happened to a riverside lot we had bought in a large village a few miles from Hamheung to start a clinic. After the flood water had receded, our lot was in the middle of a new bed the river had cut for itself through rich farmland. In other places, sand and rocks were swept onto good land and buried it.

Hundreds of families were in need of relief. The mission procured and distributed food, clothing, and bedding for the destitute.

Since many patients were now unable to pay for medical care, this seriously reduced the hospital income. The institution was at all times run as economically as possible but any reduction meant decreasing care given to those unable to pay. Soon there wasn't enough money to meet the payroll. Our staff salaries were not more than a bare cost of living at best, and some of the employees had sustained losses from the flood. The board in Canada that helped support the medical work did not permit borrowing, and it would take time to get an extra appropriation, even if the board had the money available.

After prayers one morning, I discussed the situation with the staff.

"What shall I do?" I asked. "As you all know, our income has dropped since the flood. We have to feed patients and nurses, buy medicine and supplies, and run the sterilizer and laundry, as well as pay the salaries. I see only two alternatives: reduce salaries temporarily or reduce the staff. Has anyone a better solution? What do you advise me to do?"

They looked at one another. No one said anything.

"Of course I don't want to do either, but we can't go on as we are. Shall we turn away all patients who can't pay and try to continue salaries at the present rate? What do you think I should do in this emergency?"

They looked at each other again, wondering, if anyone is dropped, who will it be?

"Reduce the salaries," some one said. There wasn't a dissenting voice. I was proud of our staff and in a few months conditions improved and the cuts were restored.

Dismissing an inefficient or irresponsible person is often a real problem. I once had to dismiss a careless orderly who, in spite of repeated instruction and reprimands, continued to disregard sterile technique which endangered the lives of patients. He and his friends pestered me for weeks, waylaying me at our gate during the day and coming to the house at night to upbraid me for my unreasonable and unjust act. Lee Sunsaing finally explained to me a way to avoid such repercussions. If the salaries of others in the same type of work were raised, he said, and that of the incompetent or offender were not, he would lose so much face he would leave. So it proved. It was rather expensive, but effective.

Loss of face is such a serious matter in the Orient that suicide may result. To commit suicide on the doorstep of the one who has offended, injured, or otherwise caused loss of face is considered an excellent way to get even. Life often is not so happy or successful that the person with a grievance, real or imagined, minds losing it and the blame of the community will rest on the person considered responsible.

An unhappy instance of this kind took place in another mission hospital where a young missionary nursing supervisor was training nurses. She was having trouble with carelessness among her students. Several babies had been burned—some severely—by uncovered hot-water bottles placed too close to them. The supervisor reprimanded the nurses responsible and lectured the class on the seriousness of this preventable accident. In spite of this, such injuries kept recurring. Finally, in desperation, the supervisor warned that if another baby was burned through such carelessness on the part of a nurse, the offending nurse would be dismissed.

A few days later, another baby was burned by an uncovered hot-water bottle and the supervisor told the nurse responsible that she must leave the hospital. The girl happened to be a member of that year's graduating class. Unable to endure the loss of face, she swallowed some tablets of mercury bichloride used for sterilizing. A short time later, another nurse found her dying in the nurses' residence.

The uproar of hospital staff, employees, and public forced

the missionary nurse to leave the country brokenhearted. All the shortcomings of the girls she was trying to train were overlooked and forgotten in the furor against the foreigner who had treated a young girl with such incredible sternness that she was forced to commit suicide. No one had a thought for the burned babies or for what kind of nurses would be produced if such carelessness were permitted. All the wrath was directed against the person who had driven a girl to take her own life.

After six years in Korea my furlough was coming due. Without Viola, who was recuperating from amoebic dysentery, Nurse Woo couldn't supervise the increasing work all alone. I'd become acquainted with a pretty young nurse in charge of the operating rooms at Severance Hospital. They generously agreed to part with her in order to help us out and I asked her to come to Hamheung. She came accompanied by her small daughter.

Nurse Lee was of medium height, with delicate features, raven black brows and hair, fair skin and rosy cheeks. She was a capable and attractive young woman who faithfully served the hospital for many years.

At the age of seventeen, her parents married her off to a man she had never seen. On her wedding day, she cried all the way in the sedan chair from her parents' home to her mother-in-law's in a village a few miles distant. As she had never been out of her home for a night in her life and hadn't even visited the next village, she felt as though she were going to a different country to live among strangers.

"Weren't you happy when you got to know them?" I asked.

"My mother-in-law was kind to me," she said.

"What did your husband do and what was he like?"

"He never did anything and I don't know what he was like."

"You don't know what your husband was like?" I exclaimed.

"No," she said. "If I met him on the street today I wouldn't know him."

"How can that be? How long did you live together?"

"It was a year before he left me, but I never once looked in his face. My mother-in-law insisted that I be modest with lowered eyes in front of my father-in-law and my husband. He never beat me, but he was rough and unkind."

When her baby came after the desertion of her husband, it was only a girl and the in-laws didn't want either of them. Though her own parents wouldn't have her back, she succeeded in persuading her mother to look after the baby while she trained as a nurse. The child, now of school age, entered Yunsaing Girls' School.

Dr. Hong was doing well in the medical department, but we needed a surgeon to do the surgical work during my year's furlough of study and promotion of the mission among the churches in Canada. Former language teacher Ahn, now a senior at Severance Medical College, recommended Dr. Koh as a competent surgeon and fine Christian man. I went to Seoul, met Dr. Koh, and engaged him to come to Hamheung. He arrived with his family a short time before I was to leave.

Dr. Koh was of middle height and like many Koreans had rather short limbs and a long body. He had a ruddy complexion, hair that stood straight up on end, and even then was showing a few white threads—unusual among Koreans of his age. He was about thirty. Dr. Koh had a hearty laugh that had an infectious quality about it. He proved to be a good surgeon with excellent judgment, a true friend, a wise counselor, and a loyal colleague.

The mission medical committee, hoping that Viola would improve faster in Canada, recommended that she go on sick leave and travel home with me when I went on furlough.

We were all packed and ready to take the noon train when an urgent call came from the hospital. I'd seen a patient the previous day and urged her to have an immediate operation. Overnight she made up her mind to have it. She insisted so strongly that I do it that I went to the hospital, scrubbed once more, and assisted Dr. Koh with the operation.

At the railway station an hour later, the patient's husband handed me a small package. It contained a dainty little silver cup and saucer which I presented to my father.

"Ahn Yung Hi Kata Osipsio" ("Go and return in peace"), chorused the crowd at the railway station to see us off.

"Remain in peace. See you next year," we called as the train pulled out. Their voices singing *God Be with You till We Meet Again* died away as the train rounded a curve and took them out of our sight.

-13-

My furlough was a happy time of reunion, visiting with family and traveling to the churches throughout Canada.

Next year, as the train approached Hamheung, I first caught a glimpse of the undulating back of the Dragon. Soon, the city came into view. When we pulled into the station a few moments later, a large delegation from the hospital staff and city churches almost overwhelmed me with the warmth of their welcome. To everyone's regret, Viola had decided it would be unwise to return and had resigned from the mission.

This time, I was assigned a room in an old brick Korean house, with its tile roof turned up at the corners in the graceful Korean style. Large polished logs supported the ceilings, and latticework formed partitions between rooms. Hot floors had been replaced by polished wood, and electric wiring and plumbing installed. A kitchen sink, running water, and a cook stove modernized the kitchen.

The Allen family from West China were living in the house. They spoke Chinese, but not Korean, so I took over the housekeeping and soon found myself involved in culinary adventures. Pak Maria, the middle-aged cook, though voluble about everything else, was reticent about her past life.

Since neither husband nor children ever appeared and were never mentioned, we supposed she was another wife cast off for failing to produce sons.

Maria never learned to count Japanese money, the currency used in Korea at that time. She continued to use the obsolete Korean monetary system of the past. On her return from market, we made up accounts. "You gave me three hundred *yang*," she would say, "and I gave one hundred *yang* for two strings of eggs and got thirty *yang* back. Now how much did I pay for the eggs?" Each item was accounted for in this way. Unable to read and write, she couldn't keep accounts, but the money she brought back always agreed with her statements. My way of housekeeping, no doubt, would scandalize a teacher of home economics, but it worked fairly well.

She seemed eager to learn to read and attended night school for three winters without achieving that result. Written recipes were useless, but her memory for them was phenomenal. If I told her how to make a cake, she could make it again ten days later. After making it twice, she remembered the recipe months later.

Unfortunately, she didn't remember other things as well. Each day after breakfast I had prayers with her and the outside man. I read a few verses of scripture and explained them simply. After two weeks of such teaching, with much repetition, Maria hadn't the remotest idea of what I had said. She went to church regularly and I often wondered what, if anything, she got out of it. I suspect it wasn't much.

Some mornings I was called to the hospital and would hurry away without giving instructions to Maria about lunch. She would shriek after me from the kitchen door, "What'll we have for lunch today?"

Sometimes I called back, "Go to McRae's, see what they're having and ask their cook how to make it. Make it for us."

Maria's successor, Chai Jung-Ine was tall and slight, her thin face dark and somber, but illuminated by her rare smile. She could read and write and keep accounts well. She too was reticent about her past life. All she ever told us was that she had gone to her mother-in-law's and returned, doubtless another cast-off wife.

Korean cooking is quite different from Western and, for a while, it was hard going on both sides. At first, when Jung-Ine started to bake something, she was likely to find there were no eggs in the pantry. Off she would go to the nearby market to buy some. Then she might find the salt dish empty and take another trip for salt. In her first week, she went to market seven times in one day, but, in a short time, she learned to plan, and one trip was sufficient. Without refrigerators in Korea's hot summers, it was necessary to get fresh food daily.

Jung-Ine thought for herself, as was evident when Ethel once ordered a shepherd's pie for the first course and an apple pie for desert. Thinking that instructions for two pies at the same meal must be a mistake, or that she had misunderstood, Jung-Ine combined them, apples in the bottom, meat and mashed potatoes on top. It was a little unusual, but quite edible. Ethel once told her to make a deep rhubarb pie with an eggcup in the middle to keep the crust from getting soggy in the juice. Since nobody could eat an eggcup, Jung-Ine knew there must be some mistake. The pie appeared without a small hump in the center where the eggcup was supposed to be. Instead, we found several slices of hard-boiled egg. Before long, Jung-Ine became a capable cook and a loyal and dear friend.

Early one cold winter morning I arrived on the night train from Wonsan, where I'd gone to treat a sick colleague. The walk of a mile from the railway station through clean snow that had fallen during the night was most refreshing after a night in the stuffy third-class sleeper.

Entering the house, I found the kitchen stove in a hundred pieces, the breakfast porridge on the ceiling, Jung-Ine covered with soot from head to foot, and blood streaming from her arms and face. Other occupants of the house in their night attire were surveying the damage. Fortunately, Jung-Ine's injuries were superficial.

The pipe from the main water supply to the hot water in

front of the stove had frozen during the night. When the cook lighted the fire in the morning, the water in the heating pipes in the fire box began to boil, but it couldn't circulate on account of the frozen pipe and mounting steam pressure blew up both pipe and stove.

Mrs. McRae invited us to breakfast and by lunchtime a discarded stove had been set up and restored to temporary use.

While I was living in the Korean house, the boxlike structure where I had spent my first few weeks in Hamheung was torn down to make way for a new Yungsaing school building. Mr. MacHattie, a missionary builder from China, designed and built both the new school and a new house for the women missionaries. As there were five of us, we needed a fairly large house. In addition to living space, it had to provide offices for Jennie Robb and Edna McLellan, who traveled among the country churches. When at home, they had numerous visitors who needed help or advice or who came out of friendliness or curiosity. Ethel, Ada, and I had our offices in the school and hospital.

Our new house was on the hill where in the early days of the mission the spirits had routed the Japanese. It was quiet except for the usual night sounds—the clang, clang, of the policeman's gong as he made his rounds and the temple bell in the next valley when the dawn streaked the sky over Dragon Hill.

We called our home the Manshun, but the married folk referred to it as the single ladies' house. We didn't spend much time there except for eating and sleeping.

The hospital had carried on very well during my absence on furlough. Now Dr. Hong went to Canada to study tuberculosis, which was still the greatest public health problem in the country. Dr. Cho came in his place and did good work for some years till he too went abroad for more training. Dr. Cho wished to continue as a surgeon, and as he was a good surgeon and a valued member of the staff, I gave him the general surgery and took over gynecology myself. I regretted giving up general surgery, but this seemed best for the work as a whole. We certainly didn't want to lose Dr. Koh.

A few days after my return, in the midst of a busy clinic one day, Kang Do-Ka interrupted to say, "*Pouine*, come out and see a sick child who's come a long way to get to our hospital. He looks bad."

Outside the door stood two lads supporting a rough home-made litter where an emaciated child was lying. The boys set down the litter and the weary travel-worn trio looked hopefully at me.

The sick lad was suffering from far-advanced tuberculosis of the spine. Pus discharged from several openings in his deformed back, and where his side and hip had been in contact with the hard floor for many painful weeks, there were large pressure sores.

"Where did you come from?" I asked.

"From Kosan," said the older lad.

"You two carried this boy all that way?"

"He's our brother. We've been walking for seven days."

About seventy miles, I thought, No wonder they look so tired.

"How did you get food and where did you sleep?"

"Every day someone gave us some rice, and most days we ate more than once, but no one would let us in. They were afraid younger brother might die in their house and his spirit haunt them. We slept outdoors, but it isn't cold now. Only our sick brother minded it."

"We'll take care of your brother in the hospital, but where will you two stay, and how will you eat?"

"I can look out for myself and my little brother," said the oldest who was thirteen, "now that younger brother'll be looked after. How long will it take for him to get well?"

"How long has he been sick?"

"A long time."

"How long? A Year?"

"More than a year."

Yum came with a stretcher and together they gently transferred the sick child to it and took him inside.

"We'll do our best for your brother," I said, "but he's been sick too long. I'm afraid he'll never be well."

The boys turned away, tears in their eyes, to find refuge in a strange city. They returned daily to see their sick brother and I soon learned their story.

Their mother died some years before and the father, unable to care for the children and earn their living too, gave them to a Buddhist priest to be brought up as acolytes. The father then went off to find work and the boys never saw or heard from him again.

For a year, they followed the monk traveling about the country with begging bowls. When the second brother lost strength and went lame, they went more slowly hoping he would recover. Instead, he became worse. After two or three months, he was quite unable to keep up with the others, and one morning they woke up in a shed to find the monk gone.

The boys then made their way back to Kosan in the hope that their father might have returned. He hadn't, and none of the villagers knew anything of him. A kindhearted friend of their father's took them in until he began to fear the sick one might die in his house. He then made the litter and sent them off on the long journey to Cheihei Hospital in Hamheung, where they heard people were admitted and treated even though they had no money.

In spite of all we could do, the child suffered much. Pain prevented sleep and the sufferer cried day and night to go home.

"Where's home?" I asked him.

"Kosan."

"What relatives have you there to take care of you?"

"Nobody."

"Then where will you stay?"

"My father's friend'll take me in."

This seemed uncertain, but the lad's constant crying to go home disturbed the other patients so much that they complained and begged that the child be sent away.

The boys agreed they should go back to Kosan. Elder Lee took them by train and stayed with them till he saw them taken in by the good neighbor who had befriended them before. How he did it I can't imagine, since he was a farmer with seven children of his own.

Two weeks later, a weary little cavalcade arrived back at the hospital. The suffering boy, soon realizing he had been better cared for there and had less pain, pleaded to be taken back. The neighbor made another litter and sent them off.

I admitted the boy again while the others fended for themselves as before. Mercifully, the sick lad's sufferings came to an end within the month.

After the funeral, the older brother said, if someone would be responsible for his nine-year-old brother, he would go to Manchuria where he heard there was work. He was thirteen and strong and could support himself, but not his little brother as well.

Many would adopt a baby or a very young child, but no one wanted a nine year old, especially one who had wandered as a beggar and never been to school. All inquiries were unavailing. No one wanted Suh Teh-Ha. Finally, in spite of much advice to the contrary, I undertook to be responsible for him. There seemed nothing else to do. This decided, the older brother left to make his way on foot to Manchuria and we lost track of him.

My new charge, Suh Teh-Ha, was a stocky, sturdy boy with well-developed muscles. His short legs never tired and could cover the ground as fast as much longer ones. He had an air of confidence that seemed to say he could look out for himself. Though he seldom spoke, his bright, dark eyes missed nothing.

Since no one in our house wanted him there, I tried to find a Korean home where he would receive loving care. Finally, my former language teacher, Ahn Sunsaing, now Dr. Ahn and practicing in Hamheung, kindly offered to take the boy into his home.

When a new baby was expected at Dr. Ahn's small house,

they needed all the space they had and I had to find another place for Teh-Ha. Lee Sunsaing, language teacher-anesthetist-secretary-purchasing agent for the hospital, took on another responsibility and the boy went to live with his family.

When I finally had Teh-Ha settled and at school, a new phase of work opened up for me with the arrival of a 1928 model Ford car. This was a gift from the young people of the United Church in Prince Edward Island. While on furlough, I drove my father's car on Nova Scotia roads, but roads and driving conditions were rather different in Korea.

Driver's licenses were difficult to obtain unless one took the Japanese police officer who gave the driving tests out to dinner several times and plied him with liquor or gave him money with which to entertain himself and his friends. I was determined not to resort to bribery.

One of the few Korean drivers in Hamheung gave me driving lessons. Driver Pak was a short, powerful, aggressive youth known, I soon found out, as the toughest character in the city. He had a vocabulary to match. His most recent exploit had been entering a neighbor's house through a hole he dug in the mud wall and stealing a young bride who happened to be alone for the evening. He allowed her to go home the next day, but husband and family refused to have her back. This I learned much later.

Driving through the street market, Pak took the wheel himself. Country people brought their produce one day in five and displayed it in the streets. Except in the cow market, women did most of the buying and selling—and expert bargainers they were. They carried their goods on their heads for miles, often leaving home before daylight and getting back after dark. Half of them had babies on their backs—children too young to be left home because they had to be nursed during the day. Spread in the streets were rakes, hoes, harrows, wooden clogs, utensils, straw ropes, straw shoes, brooms, paper fans, oiled paper covers for horsehair hats, the hats themselves, and cases for them. Another section displayed strings of eggs wrapped in straw, live chickens, vegetables, fish, grain, and various kinds of fruit in season.

Menders of shoes and crockery plied their trades while, with a huge tray of candy covered with sesame seed suspended from his sturdy shoulders, the candy seller pushed his way through the crowd, with his big scissors clattering to announce his approach. Bull cart drivers shouting *Soolgy, soolgy,* "cart, cart," seemed about to crush the piles of eggs and overturn the buckets of red peppers in their way, but miraculously everything was snatched aside in time. People moved back into the center of the street the moment the vehicle passed.

On approaching this maelstrom, Pak blew his horn constantly, but no one paid any attention. The car had to stop. There was more blowing, then Pak shouted abuse. This failing, he got out and laid about him lustily with his heavy fists. People with their wares moved back just far enough for the car to get by. Meanwhile, I sat helpless in the vehicle noting with dismay the outraged expressions on the faces of the market folk so roughly treated, who, I feared, thought the driver was doing my bidding.

The first part of the driving test consisted in guiding an old wreck of a car that looked and sounded as though it might fall to pieces during the ordeal around a maze constructed of ropes fastened to posts. Another foreigner was ordered to use his own car for the test, while I was not permitted to use mine. This man declared that his long car couldn't possibly get around without touching the ropes. No doubt he was right, and no doubt that was why he had to use it. The first touch disqualified him.

I had practiced in the maze, and as a result, managed to pass that part of the test. Then the officer conducting the examination ordered me to drive out of the city and turn around on a narrow road only two feet wider than the car, with rice fields deep in mud and water on both sides, easy enough to slip into. But getting out would be another story. I gave up, unwilling to try what I felt I couldn't do, and so failed the test given only once in six months.

When next I tried, I thought I'd passed, but weeks went by and the license was never granted. Korean friends said all that was needed was to send a generous sum to the policeman and the license would be forthcoming. This didn't appeal to me, and I tried a third time six months later, and at last got my license.

Driving was always an adventure. Roads were narrow, crooked, unpaved. Floods in the rainy season washed away bridges and, if after the rains were past, a bus or truck could ford the river, it didn't seem necessary to replace a missing bridge. Over small streams and irrigation canals, the villagers themselves often removed the bridges to prevent their loss during the rains. Fording streams and negotiating the banks of canals were a part of every car journey outside the city.

Some bridges consisted of only two lines of boards laid lengthwise on the crosspieces. On such an open-work bridge high above a river, driving was an exciting experience. Edna McLellan accompanied by another missionary once drove over such a bridge—a long one and not altogether straight—with her passenger walking backward on the boards ahead of the car to help Edna keep on the track. After a nerve-racking few minutes, realizing she was almost across, Edna relaxed and gave the car more gas. It took a sudden spurt forward and, to avoid being run over, the woman on the bridge had to drop through. Fortunately, she escaped the rocks and fell in the water ten feet below. She had a wet cold ride for the remaining miles to their destination.

There were neither filling nor service stations. Truck and bus companies starting up in the city did their own servicing. The only way we could get repairs done was by hiring a driver on his day off, if we could find one willing to do the work. I knew the anatomy of the Ford and could change a tire and connect up the battery when the jolting had disconnected it, but I had neither knowledge nor tools to do much more.

Fortunately, Korean drivers never passed anyone in trouble. They invariably stopped to help. One Sunday morning after rounds in the hospital, Elder Lee, some nurses, and I started for the country where we were due to visit a church and see a patient. I had had the car checked over the previous day. We were scarcely out of the city when without warning the front left side took a sudden dip and the wheel jumped across the ditch and rolled away across the fields on an expedition of its own. Because the road was bad, we were going so slowly I stopped the car at once and the passengers weren't even shaken up.

While I was pursuing the runaway wheel, the driver of an approaching bus saw what had happened and reached the wheel before I did. Within ten minutes, three buses and a truck were lined up on the side of the road while the drivers jacked up my car and replaced the wheel. We were all soon on our way again; my benefactors refused anything but thanks. Even that, they said in the expressive Korean idiom, was a thousand times ten thousand words too many.

Once after finding a trip longer than expected, I discovered the gasoline getting low and tried to buy some at a bus station. The Japanese in charge refused, saying it was illegal to sell the company supply, and no doubt he was right. I then asked to borrow a five-gallon tin, promising to replace it by the next trip of the bus. Again he refused with quite unnecessary abuse. A Korean driver intervening on my behalf was roundly cursed for it. Without a word, he went inside, brought out a five-gallon tin, and emptied it into my tank. I replaced the gas on the next bus trip and hoped the sympathetic driver didn't lose his job for his helpfulness.

The only time I ever had any unpleasantness with Koreans on the roads was while returning from a nearby town where I had gone to see a patient. It was market day and I overtook a line of about thirty bull carts on their way home. Local bull carts were distinctive in having a stout piece of wood projecting about a foot beyond the sides of the heavily built cart. Drivers saw no reason to pull to the side for a car, for on narrow roads those projections were quite a hazard for motorists. They could make a big dent in the car body without suffering any damage themselves.

It was usually quite a feat to pass a line of carts because

they never observed any rule of the road—if they knew of any—some taking one side, some the other, if they moved off the middle at all. A car had to wind its way from one side of the road to the other among them.

Nearing the line of carts, I blew the horn hoping that some at least might pull over. Some driver must recently have annoyed these carters for they had evidently agreed to make trouble for the next one who happened along. All stayed in the middle of the narrow road blocking it completely. In half a mile, I hadn't passed one cart, and the men were laughing and calling to one another not to let me pass. As I still had several miles to go, at this rate, it would be late before I got back and I had rounds to make in the hospital, and I worried that some emergency case might be waiting for me.

I knew a bus would be along soon and the carts would have to make way for it. I meant to follow it closely and get by before the carters could block the road again. This worked, and the men were so angry they cursed loudly.

It was fun picking up people on the road.

Overtaking an old couple carrying heavy loads one day, I said, "*Yung Kam*" (old man, being a respectful way in our province to address an elderly man), "won't you have a ride? Your loads are heavy."

"We've no money," replied the man and the old couple trudged on.

"I don't take money. There's room in the car and you must be tired. I'd like to give you a lift. Where are you going?"

"To Pukchudong. Thank you. Thank you. Where was there ever such kindness as this?"

They climbed in and sat down, the old man still bent forward under his load while his wife lowered hers from her head to her lap.

"Set your loads down," I urged. "You needn't carry them now."

"It's enough for you to take *us* in the automobile and we can't think of letting you carry our loads too."

"That's all right," I said smiling. "The car doesn't mind and your loads will get there as soon as you do."

With the loads set down, the passengers relaxed to enjoy their first car ride.

"Won't we have a story to tell in the village tonight," said the woman.

"Won't we indeed! Just look at the fields fly by! This thing goes as fast as the train."

"That's our village there," said the man, pointing to a group of straw thatched mud houses at the foot of a steep hill a mile away across the rice fields. "Can you stop this thing?"

I stopped the car, and with many bows and farewells, the couple adjusted their loads on head and back and set out for their village.

The most amusing, though exasperating, experience while driving occurred on a narrow street in Hamheung where a mentally deranged youth roamed who imagined himself a motorcar. Whenever he met a brother car, he conceived it his duty to greet and embrace it.

The only way to get through a narrow street was to keep the horn going to clear the way of pedestrians. This also brought out the human "car," who took his place, arms extended, in the center of the street. The car had to stop when the misguided fellow climbed on the hood and honked back. There was no use pulling him off as he climbed on again while I was getting back in. There was nothing to do but sit there helplessly and join in the laughter of the crowd who quickly collected to see the fun. When they'd had enough, they removed the unfortunate boy and held him till I got away.

In villages, cars were such a rarity that when we went for a church service, public health meeting, or to see a patient, someone had to guard the vehicle. No villager would steal anything or willingly disable the car; but children out of curiosity and ignorance would experiment, often running down the battery by turning on the lights, which by law had to be turned on from outside, or by letting the air out of the tires. Of course, they generally forgot to replace the cap.

One night when we were holding a meeting in a village to which there was no road, we left the Ford locked on the highway. It was a very dark night and we thought no one would be on the road. On returning a couple of hours later, the lock was gone, the door open, and a box of tracts and Bibles missing. It would have been interesting to see the faces of the thieves when they opened the box. Fortunately, they didn't look under the seat and so missed the tools which no doubt were what they were after.

Elder Lee never learned what was a reasonable load for the vehicle. Once when I had to cross the railway and ford a brook to get back on the highway after a village meeting, I asked him and Nurse Woo to cross by themselves while I maneuvered the railway embankment and the stream unencumbered.

Back on the road, a torrent of children poured in at the four doors; the body sank lower till it was resting heavily on the axles and not another child could possibly squeeze in. After some had done their best and failed to enter, a child inside said: "All right now, let's go."

"What's all this?" I demanded. "We can't go with this many. I can't move hand or foot to drive and the car won't carry us all. Besides, other people are coming to go with me. You'll all have to get out."

"We've never had a car ride in our lives," they chorused, "and Elder Lee said you'd take us."

"I can't take all of you. Some will have to get out. Now scram."

No one moved.

"I'm not going one foot till some of you get out," I said firmly.

Very reluctantly, about six did.

"We can't go yet. More will have to get out."

After another unwilling exodus, the chassis rose from the axles and I drove carefully about three miles to the next village, disgorged fifteen children aged about nine to fourteen, and went back for my original passengers.

"Lee Changno," I remonstrated when they were aboard, "how did that avalanche of children come to descend on me like that?"

"They'd never had a car ride, and I knew you'd be glad to make them happy."

"So I would, in reasonable numbers, but to drive with that many was impossible. I couldn't move and the car might break down." The elder wasn't impressed.

"Who'd ever think a thing made of iron would be as weak as that," he murmured skeptically.

Now that transportation was quick and easy, we held meetings in village churches for Gospel talks and health instruction. In summer, farmers worked from dawn to dark, then had supper, and often were too weary to do anything but go to sleep afterward. If they came it would not be till nine o'clock or later. Children would be there in swarms. After teaching them a song, telling Bible stories, and giving a simple health talk, we tried to send them home. It didn't work. No child would leave. By the time the adult meeting was half over, the youngsters were either restless or asleep, but to go home before they saw a moving car was unthinkable.

Such meetings were held in the church or the church grounds since no village had a public hall and the use of schools for such purposes was not permitted. Small churches were crowded to the doors, with people leaning in the windows. Usually, there were too many for the church and the meeting would be held outdoors. If the weather were not too cold, the Christians would spread straw mats from their houses on the frozen ground in the churchyard for people to sit on. We suspended a large sheet from one corner of the church to that of the next house and set up our projector on the box we brought our equipment in. Though the picture on the sheet was slightly less brilliant than one on a proper projector screen, this was compensated for by the audience being able to view the pictures from both sides. People came from surrounding villages and we often had an audience of several hundred.

Elder Lee would tell a Bible story while I ran the projector. His local touches brought the ancient stories right up-to-date.

"Look," he would cry as the picture of the prodigal son returning home to his father appeared on the sheet. "Look at the foolish son now! His fine silk robe pawned, his horsehair hat gone, his money wasted with *kesaings* and liquor. He's filthy, in rags, the smell of the pigs on him. The foolish young rich man who wouldn't listen to his old father became a beggar.

"Look! His father sees him coming and runs to meet him. He doesn't care that the money is gone, he doesn't care for the rags and the smell of the pigs, he cares only for his lost son who's come back to him. God is like that. He cares for us though we've left him like the foolish son did. All we have to do to go to him is to say, like the son in the picture, 'I've sinned. Please forgive me,' and God will meet us and take us into his house. Is there somebody here tonight who wants to give up the old ways and be God's son?"

And always there was. The deacons welcomed each who put up a hand and found out where he or she lived in order to visit and encourage him.

Then came public health pictures and talk. Slides from abroad were of little use. A picture of a woman going to the clinic for prenatal care evoked the response, "Those foreigners must be pretty weak if they have to go to see a doctor for a thing like a baby coming. Our women are much stronger."

One evening I gave a talk on typhoid fever, which was always present and caused numerous deaths every year. Describing how flies frequent filthy places and carry the bacilli of disease on their legs and feet to the kitchen and the food, I showed a picture of a fly magnified to impressive dimensions on the screen. I urged people to keep food covered, to kill flies, and described safe ways to dispose of filth and night soil. As I was gathering up my equipment after the meeting, I heard some women discussing what they had seen and heard.

"If flies in Western countries are that big," said one, "no wonder foreigners are afraid of them, but our little Korean flies wouldn't hurt anybody."

I was deflated. In Korea, humility is forced on one.

On another occasion, a cheeky youth said he had a question to ask. He asked it right off: "Why haven't women got whiskers?" People pricked up their ears and some snickered. I replied there wasn't time to explain that now but if he cared to come to the hospital next day I'd be pleased to enlighten him. Of course, he never came.

Nurses made more effective speakers in the villages than doctors who were inclined to use scientific terms that were over the heads of the audience. Nurses used the language of the village women and were understood. Nurse Woo was one of the most effective speakers I ever heard.

These visits were an encouragement to the small groups of Christians carrying on without trained leaders and helped them and others realize that Jesus's teaching was not merely for Sunday, saving souls, and life after death, but was also concerned with improving life, health, and living conditions for people in their own communities here and now. Those who failed to understand or accept the spiritual message of the church usually appreciated the health program.

There were always some who came for free medical advice. Sometimes it was simple to do or give what was needed. Serious cases we urged to go to the Cheihei Hospital, and many did who probably would not have without the personal contact in the village.

The local church leader would close the meeting with a brief prayer of thanks for the teachers who had come to their village that night, after which Elder Lee would ask God's blessing on them all, especially those who had just decided to be his followers.

Elder Lee died not long ago, old and nearly blind, respected by all who heard of him, loved by all who knew him.

He was a gentleman of old Korea who never quite adjusted to modern ways. But he served his Lord faithfully from the time he first heard of him in his youth, through all his days, and death for him was the gate of heaven.

-14-

Between terms at language school, Ada Sandell had been giving valuable assistance with the nursing in the hospital. When she finished her course, she plunged full time into the work. On account of the many nursing problems with family attendants and untrained nursing aids, together with the impossibility of getting educated girls to work in a hospital, the mission in 1928 decided to start a training school for nurses with Ada as principal.

Although hospital work was generally considered menial labor, there was still a great desire for education and few opportunities. We hoped that parents might be willing for their daughters graduating from elementary school to continue their education in a school of nursing where they would receive a diploma on graduation and have a job waiting for them. This proved to be the case. Apparently a student in a school—any kind of a school—was quite different from a girl working in a hospital.

On my return from furlough that year, I accepted two bright girls from among several who applied to enter the infant school of nursing. They were graduates of the six-year elementary-school course. One soon dropped out to be married. Next year we accepted two others, one of them the granddaughter of Kang Do-Ka. To supplement their education, we had to teach some subjects not usually included in a Western course of nursing. These girls had to know Japanese to take the government examination for registration. They had to have more mathematics, some elementary chemistry, and since there were few medical terms in Korean, they had to learn them in English. Lee Sunsaing taught Korean and Japanese; the doctors instructed in anatomy and medical subjects; I taught physiology and English; and when Ada came, she taught nursing arts and supervised the nursing in clinic and wards.

Some parents who gave grudging permission for their daughters to enter the school had reservations. One mother who came to visit her daughter met Miss Sandell in the corridor and accosted her with, "Where's that girl of mine? Carrying a bedpan around somewhere I suppose?"

"No," said Ada who happened to be carrying one herself at the moment. "No, she isn't. She's studying in the classroom."

After three months study, the student nurses began to help a little on the wards, by assisting graduate nurses Miss Woo and Mrs. Lee. The nurses appreciated the help and the novices enjoyed both the contact with patients and the feeling of being useful.

At first, the girls found it difficult to accept responsibility, and holidays were not happy occasions. Why couldn't they all have the whole day off? How could one be expected to stay on duty while another was away having a good time?

After six months study and probation, they passed their tests satisfactorily and were accepted—no longer probationers—but regular student nurses. At a dignified and impressive ceremony, they received their nurses' caps. People began to see that nurses were not only respectable but worthy members of the community, who provided capable and needed services to the sick. However, there were still hurdles to be overcome.

Night duty was something never heard of before. As no

other hospital provided nursing care at night, our students didn't see why they should have to do such an unprecedented thing. Ada put in many weary hours at night to help and encourage them. One night she asked Yum Ke-Moon, who was on duty in the men's wards, why the girls were so scared of night duty.

"What can you expect?" he replied. "The mission built the hospital on a piece of property that has always been known to harbor evil spirits. That's why Mr. McRae was able to buy it. Then you put young girls on night duty. Why wouldn't they be afraid?"

She asked Yum if he believed there were evil spirits around at night. His reply was, "Of course."

Eventually the student nurses seemed to lose their fear and to accept night duty as a part of their training and responsibility, though they were never really happy about it and never adjusted properly to it. Instead of sleeping through the day, they insisted on getting up and having all the meals with the day nurses. Thus, they never got enough sleep when on night duty and one week was all they could take at a time.

When a new minister in the lower church was invited to the hospital Christmas celebration, the staff provided the program. The nurses took several parts, including a chorus and play. Reverend Mr. Kim was impressed. In thanking me for inviting him, he repeated in obvious surprise, "These nurses are *nice* girls, *really* nice girls."

"Of course they are," I told him. "What did you think they'd be like?"

"I didn't know nurses were like that. They're fine girls."

Afterward, when announcing in church the date of examination for entrance to the school of nursing, that minister added his personal advice. He recommended parents to take advantage of this opportunity to give their daughters nurse's training.

Though the Cheihei Hospital infant school of nursing gave a full three-year course it wasn't recognized by the government. Government approved two different courses, one year for midwives and a two-year course for nurses. Our course included both.

Under government rules, a girl could become a registered nurse by studying at home and passing the examination without ever having been inside the door of a hospital or having any practical experience whatever. Many Japanese nurses obtained their licenses that way. Korean students had to take their government examinations in Japanese—a foreign language. Though they had had a three-year course with good practical training and experience, they usually failed the examination one or more times, while Japanese girls with no bedside training or experience succeeded. Our students considered this discrimination and resented it deeply. They had our sympathy, but we could do nothing about it without resorting to bribery.

Another difficulty was that the young girls felt it impossible to give regular nursing care to men patients. The girls were too modest and feared they would be criticized if they did. The solution was to train men. We trained four, three of whom proved to be capable and reliable male nurses, a valuable addition to the nursing staff. Some other hospitals, learning of the good work done by our male nurses, engaged some of them.

One girl, a high school graduate, after the course started, found herself studying with middle school graduates. This was too much for her with her superior education and she dropped out. However, one or two classes later, nursing had acquired such a reputation that more high school graduates applied and we were able to raise the standards for matriculation, and thus improve the status of nurses in the eyes of the public.

The daughter of a man on whom I operated for a complication of tuberculosis came to the hospital with her father to nurse him. She was so interested in seeing the three young girls in the first class and observing their work that the next year she entered the new class of five and proved one of the best of the seventy-five or so nurses who graduated during the years from our small school of nursing.

Ada or I, and often both of us, made rounds at night to see the patients and to send away surplus visitors hoping to spend the night by hiding under the beds or sleeping in any they found unoccupied.

The first graduation in 1932 was a happy occasion. The ceremony was held in the lower church where friends and relatives could all attend. They all came. A choir of nurses gave a special school song written for the event. The three new graduates stood and repeated the solemn words of the Florence Nightingale pledge.

> "I solemnly pledge myself before God and in the presence of this assembly, to pass my life in purity, and to practise my profession faithfully. With loyalty will I endeavor to aid the physician in his work, and devote myself to the welfare of those committed to my care."

Next morning when the new graduates came on duty with black bands on their caps, wearing their graduates' pins, the whole hospital cheered them. The next year there were five graduates. Graduate nurses as they became available replaced the former nursing aids, with the result that the nursing service of the hospital was immensely improved.

An early graduate, Lee Ahn-Soon, a tall rosy-cheeked, fine-looking girl, especially interested in the operating room and surgical work, was so proficient at it that she was soon given charge of that department. After a year, her family arranged a marriage for her. She didn't know the prospective groom and didn't want to be married, but girls obeyed their parents and "she was sent to her mother-in-law's." This common expression explains the state of affairs well, for the bride marries the whole family, particularly the mother-in-law, and often sees much more of her than of her husband.

This mother-in-law was not at all sure a nurse's training

was an asset to anybody. She decided to test her new daughter-in-law to see what she could do. When the older woman saw one of the household fowls in distress, she told Ahn-Soon to attend to it. The girl found the greedy bird had got into the grain, gorged itself, then drunk water. Ahn-Soon made the diagnosis at once. The grain in the hen's crop swelled, distending it greatly. The poor thing couldn't get the grain up or down.

The nurse was equal to the occasion. She hadn't worked in the operating room for nothing. She shaved off the feathers over the crop, cleansed the area, and painted it with antiseptic. While she was doing this, a knife, needle, thread, and a pair of scissors were boiling over the *wharro,* "charcoal brazier," found in every Korean kitchen.

With capable fingers, Ahn-Soon quickly incised the skin, opened the crop, scooped out the swollen grain, and sewed up the wound neatly in layers. The fowl was obviously relieved, the wound healed promptly, and, at least in that family, the reputation of the Cheihei Hospital School of Nursing was made.

Some months later, I was called to that house to help the young wife have her baby. The old-fashioned mother-in-law had refused to let her have prenatal care. *She* had never seen a doctor before *her* babies were born and she'd had six. She forgot to mention that three of them had died in infancy—a common fate—for which it never occurred to her that she might in any way be responsible.

Ahn-Soon went into labor at home and after many hours the mother-in-law finally realized the young mother was having an unusually hard time. When they sent for me, I found she was about to have twins.

Trying to keep hands and gown sterile while sprawling around on the floor is neither simple nor easy. When the source of light is a single candle or even a twenty-five candle power electric bulb suspended just below the ceiling in a partition between two rooms, the illumination near the floor is anything but adequate.

Twin boys soon greeted the world with lusty cries. The father modestly said nothing but his eyes shone, the grandparents were jubilant, and the weary young mother said she would have been contented with one.

A year later, during a busy morning in the clinic, Nurse Woo interrupted to announce with distress in her eyes, "Ahn-Soon's on a stretcher at the door and she looks like death."

Hastening out, I met her being carried in and she *did* look like death. She was gasping for breath and unable to speak, and the pleading look in her dark eyes. I reached for her pulse and the look of confidence she gave me as her fingers closed on mine smote me to the heart, as I saw she was beyond hope of recovery.

When she became pregnant again, her husband said he didn't want another troublesome brat in the house till the twins were older and insisted she have an abortion. She objected as she didn't want to lose her baby and she knew that induced abortions outside a hospital were dangerous. Against her will, her husband brought a young doctor friend of his to the house to perform the operation.

Infection followed and the husband, ashamed of his folly, refused to take her to the hospital until too late. This was before the days of antibiotics. Sulfa drugs had just come on the market and we had been able to get some sulfanilamide, the first available and not as effective as later sulfa drugs were. We used it freely, but the young mother, another victim of ignorance, died before it had time to take effect.

Wives come cheap, and it didn't take long to get a replacement.

Another of our usually bright and cheerful student nurses suddenly became unaccountably depressed, frequently bursting into tears without obvious cause.

"Are you sick, Chungie?" asked Ada coming on the girl leaning on a desk with her hand on her arms.

"No," she replied.

"Then what's the matter? Can we do anything about it?"

Chungie gave no answer but a sob.

"Is someone sick or in trouble at home?"

"No. Nothing's wrong." And she sobbed harder.

It was useless to try to force a confidence, but one of Chungie's classmates explained. There were only girls in Chungie's family and several years had passed since the last had been born. The father decided something had to be done to get a son. He wasn't well enough off to support two households and so was about to bring a concubine to live with the family, and they were upset about it.

The concubine came and the "big" wife made the best of the situation, but couldn't quite resist the temptation to order the "little" wife around enough to let her know who was boss. The younger woman understood and accepted her position. The nurse's tears soon disappeared and the household, if not exactly content, has at least become resigned to the situation.

When in due time the hoped-for son arrived, the legal wife appeared as pleased and fond of the boy as his own mother. When he was sick, both women brought him to the hospital together, one as likely as the other to have him on her back. Sometimes I wondered if the little fellow really knew which woman was his mother.

Of the seventy-five who graduated from the school of nursing, most soon married and were better wives and mothers for the training they received in the hospital. They gave community service, privately or in hospitals, while those who lived outside the city often sent or brought patients for treatment. They came themselves for prenatal care, which set a good example to other young mothers who didn't know that this was a wise thing to do. If they lived near enough, they came to the hospital to have their babies, giving a good demonstration to those who thought hospitals were only places for the dying. They taught Sunday school, sang in the choir, and were leaders in the women's evangelist society. In these ways, our nurses exerted a fine influence for public health and the Christian cause wherever they lived.

Their training in care of tuberculosis and its prevention began to reach the families of sufferers from that dread disease. Many came to the hospital for examination and to start treatment, and, encouraged by the nurses, continued it at home.

During those years in South Hamkyung province, nursing rose in public esteem from a despised occupation fit only for those who would otherwise starve, to a respected vocation second only to that of teacher. Indeed, many of our nurses out in the community soon came to be addressed as teacher, a title that formerly no one would have thought of bestowing on a nurse.

After the communist takeover in the North, some of these nurses escaped to the South. Most lost their diplomas and registration in their flight. Years after they graduated, they took the nursing examination over again in the South along with nurses fresh from their studies at large schools of nursing who had higher matriculation requirements. The older women from Cheihei Hospital passed the examinations and received new licenses and registration in the South.

During the Korean War, there were many thousands of refugees and one hundred eighty thousand prisoners of war on Koje Island off Korea's south coast. Among the refugees were some from Hamheung. I visited them on a country road near the prisoner of war camp and met one of our early graduate nurses. She was dressed in a nondescript array of garments from relief packages. On recognizing one another, we rushed into each other's arms and laughed and cried together.

She didn't know that any missionaries had been able to get back to Korea or where they were if they had. I didn't know where any of our nurses were, what hardships they had endured, or who had managed to survive. My former student's husband and oldest son had got across the line to freedom, but the old people and younger children were unable to take the long walk through the snow-covered mountains. They had to keep away from the roads, hide by day, and travel at night. There was no word of the fate of those left in the North. Nor did they have any way of learning the fate of the ones who had fled.

"What are you doing here?" I asked. "How are you managing to live?"

"I'm chief nurse at the prisoner of war hospital," she said. "I have three thousand patients to care for. After seeing the terrible deeds of the communists, I didn't think I *could* nurse one of them, but these lads are just homesick and wounded Korean boys. They call me Mother and I look after them just like I would my lost children."

-15-

One beautiful summer morning three missionaries with a group of Korean church people took the train north from Hamheung about seventy miles to Samho on Korea's rugged eastern coast. The old church in Samho had been outgrown and we went to attend the dedication of a new one. From the train we caught glimpses of the rocky coastline of the Sea of Japan, which Koreans called the East Sea, where spray dashed wildly at the foot of dark precipices. On the west, green fields were interspersed with gnarled pines whose lower branches had been cut off for fuel; the mountains dipped into the valleys. The glorious day made one happy to be alive. It was good, too, to get away from the sights and sad tales of unnecessary suffering in the hospital.

The chief contributor to the new church was a well-to-do man in middle life who, on account of his ability and integrity, had become the headman of three districts. This was an unheard of position for a Korean under the Japanese. He was now an elder in the church, and as there were many Elder Kim's in the country, he was known as Samho Kim Changno.

When, fifteen years before, the early Korean Christians began to preach in Samho, he had vigorously opposed the new religion and stood up for the continuance of the worship of the honorable ancestors. However, several villagers had become Christians in spite of him and began to hold worship in their own houses. Before long, there were too many Christians to meet in a house and, much against the headman's wishes, they built themselves a small mud church.

On the day of the dedication of the church, he was so angry that, though not usually a drinking man, he got drunk to drown his feelings of annoyance. During the morning, seeing crowds of people going to the church and hearing the singing from within, he decided to go and see what was going on.

The Christians welcomed him warmly and conducted him to the most prominent place in front of the pulpit. The headman liked the singing, found the words from the Book were very strange, but the sermon was clear and understandable and he heard nothing he could object to. Having seen enough, he wanted to leave again, but was ashamed to walk from his place so far in front, especially as he feared his gait might not be quite steady.

When he heard that *Hananim,* "the Great Spirit," had sent His son into the world to show mankind that He loved and cared for them, his heart was touched. There was nothing like that in the teachings of Confucius. All through the week he couldn't forget what he had heard, and next Sunday he went again to the church.

He decided to believe, and to him that meant action. Gathering his family together, he told them that from now on they were all Christians and must behave as such. He sent to Hamheung to buy Bibles and hymnbooks for each member of his household and brought a man from the city to teach them to sing. He wrote to his oldest son at the university in Tokyo telling him that he too, from now on, must be a Christian.

The son replied that he had been a Christian for sometime, but was afraid to tell his father.

The father asked for instruction in the new faith and learned among other things that Christians were not to have more than one wife. Samho Kim was well able to afford more than one and, indeed, had three.

The idea of losing any of them was quite a shock. All of them had children and he couldn't think of sending a mother away from her children or letting any of his children go away with the mother. However, having set out to be a Christian, he was resolved to go the whole way.

"Well," he said to Pastor Cho who was instructing him, "if I have to do it, I will. I'll send the old one away. I never did care a great deal for her anyway. The second one isn't much of a housekeeper and I can get along without her, but the third one I picked out for myself and she's the youngest and prettiest, so I'll keep her."

"But," said the pastor, "the first is the legal wife and the others only concubines. You must keep the legal wife."

Here was a pretty pass. Just because he'd become a Christian his home was to be broken up. Was it worth it?

He wouldn't go back on his word. He kept his first wife and sent the others away, well provided for, and soon they had new homes.

At the railway station, we found a welcoming crowd from the village waiting to escort us across the hills and along the beach to Samho.

"We're going to walk across the crying sands," they told me.

"Crying sand! What do you mean?"

"The sand on our beach here at Samho cries out as though it were being hurt when anyone walks on it. There are only two places in all Korea where the sand cries and Samho is one of them."

This seemed strange but, sure enough, when we came to the beach there was a creaking squeaking sound from the sand at every step, a sound I've never heard on any other beach.

As we approached the village, we saw the fine new brick church beside the old one on a hilltop where it made a landmark from land or sea.

There was special music, a dedicatory prayer, and a sermon by a visiting Korean pastor. Then came congratulatory speeches until the children became restless and the women began to slip out to see to the dinner that was served to all. Foreigners sitting cross-legged on the floor began to stretch their legs to get sensation back before attempting to rise.

A sumptuous dinner of rice, soup, meat, and various kinds of delicious fish with other delicacies was served in the old church where doors from several houses had been placed on boxes to serve as tables.

After dinner, we went to the shore to see the fishing boats and were taken for a sail in one. We landed on a large rock in the harbor where there was no soil whatever. A few lichens grew on the bare rock, as well as a strange plant I've never seen anywhere else. A rosette of pale green fleshy leaves clung without roots to the surface of the rock and raised a single six-inch spike topped with small white flowers.

"This plant," said one of the elder's sons accompanying us, "not only lives and grows without soil or roots, but it will survive and keep fresh for months hanging up in the dry air of a house. This kind of plant is found in only a few places."

I took some home and hung them on a line in the kitchen where suspended in the air they not only lived, but grew a little during the next six months.

Some of the guests took the evening train home, but we spent the night in the elder's house. Next morning, at dawn, we counted seventy fishing boats setting out for the day's work, with sails flashing in the morning sun—a lovely sight.

Before we finished a breakfast of rice, soup, and fish with the kimche which appears at every Korean meal, the sick began to arrive and the clinic started. The sons of the household acted as nurses and secretaries, by taking down names, addresses, diagnoses, and my recommendations for treatment. When we left on the afternoon train, one son accompanied us to Hamheung to bring back the medicines he would distribute to the patients.

I can never forget the kindness and fellowship of those fishers and farmers, nor recall those days without sadness, for two of the elder's fine sons were later murdered by the communists for being Christians. Others failed to escape from the North and their fate is unknown. The old elder, fortunately for him, reached his Father's house in peace before the terrors of war fell upon his country and family. Two sons escaped to the South where one is a leader in the church as was his father before him. The other is now pastor of a Korean congregation in Canada.

Country villages were not the only places where the church was progressing. In Hamheung, the two city churches grew until they felt strong enough to divide and start another in a section of the city without a church. Leaders from the two congregations who lived in the new district were appointed to help start the new church; others helped too until there were enough new Christians to carry on by themselves.

One of the most diligent workers in the lower church was a tiny bundle of energy by the name of Koong *Chipsa*, "Deaconess" Koong. Being a grandmother, she wasn't expected to work any more and so was free to give all her time to the church. This she did with enthusiasm.

On Saturdays, she visited any members who weren't in the habit of attending regularly to remind them that next day would be Sunday and to invite them to the services. She called on members of the women's group and, if any failed to appear on Sunday, she went around on Monday to inquire about their health and collect their pledged offering. The sick were her special care and, if anyone needed help in any way, Deaconess Koong could be counted on to give it.

On a visit to a relative in a village six miles from the city she inquired about the church and to her great distress heard it had closed.

The little old lady, a look of determination in her bright eyes, asked for the key of the church and a broom. She swept down the cobwebs, opened the windows, and swept the floor. Then she sat down in the clean church and prayed that soon there would again be a congregation worshiping there.

On her way home she came to the hospital and asked me

to send the hospital evangelist regularly to that village.

"Do you think there's anyone there ready to believe?" I asked. "If they were at all interested, wouldn't they have become Christians while the church was among them?"

"They can't believe unless someone preaches to them and teaches them and until there's a congregation there to give them encouragement and help."

"Do send someone," pleaded Koong *Chipsa*. "I'm going to get volunteers from our women's group to walk out there early on Sunday mornings to gather up the people. You *will* send somebody, won't you?"

When I presented this request to the hospital evangelistic team, they offered to walk to their churches several miles distant so the car could take Elder Lee to the village with the closed church. Koong *Chipsa* had no difficulty getting women to walk with her the six miles to collect a congregation. The women went and so did Elder Lee, till there was again a little group to worship in that village.

About the same time, a very conservative village on the plain across the river objected when a few of their young people wanted to become Christians. The older folk announced that no preaching and no Christians would be tolerated there.

"It's too bad," said Elder Lee telling me this. "Something should be done to help those young people."

"All right. Let's have a meeting there so people can hear for themselves whether what is said is good or bad."

"They say they won't allow a Christian meeting."

"Let's go anyway and see what happens."

So we loaded the car with members of the preaching team and went.

As expected, a crowd had gathered and were a bit noisy. The elder and others of our party slipped away in the dark and confusion and held worship with the new Christians in one of their houses, while I stayed by the car and drew the attention of the villagers. A few stones were thrown to register dissatisfaction, but not with the intention of hurting anyone. I talked to some of the women nearest me. They were friendly enough and asked why I came to their country.

"I heard there weren't enough doctors in Korea and I came to see if I could help."

"That's right," said someone from the crowd. "I know her. She's the superintendent of the Cheihei Hospital and she operated on my mother when everyone said she was going to die. This foreigner operated on her and saved her life. We should be proud she came to our village."

There was no trouble then or afterward and within a year there were enough Christians in that village to build themselves a little church.

The changed lives of the Christians were as effective as preaching.

Testimony to Christian living came at times from unexpected sources. At a meeting in the local Japanese government office, headmen from all the districts in the county in which Hamheung is located reported on conditions and problems in their areas.

The headman from Pukchudong, a non-Christian, arose in his turn and said he thought he had the best district in the country. He had no problems. There were no thieves. A man could leave his plow in the field and it would be there in the morning. One might forget to lock the gate at night, but nothing would be missing next day.

"That *is* a strange state of affairs," said the official. "No wonder you say you have the best district in the county. How do you account for it?"

"Nearly everybody in Pukchudong is a Christian," replied the headman. "That accounts for it."

Not only did the idea of God as the Great Spirit seem natural to those who believed in many local spirits, but Bible narratives and parables with their Oriental setting are more real to Koreans than to those with Western backgrounds.

The story of the starving Lazarus at the rich man's gate is familiar in a country where beggars gather for the leavings from every dinner party. The outcast leprosy patient whom everyone shuns is well-known to all. There is no commoner sight than the woman at the village well with her water jar.

"Let me first bury my father," the excuse given by a man whom Jesus called to follow him is still pertinent in Korea.

"We're glad to have you come to church," said Elder Lee to a man who had been attending for some time. "You've learned a lot about God and Jesus. Wouldn't you like to become a Christian?"

"Yes, I would, and I mean to some day, but not until after my father has left the world. It would break his heart to think I wouldn't worship his spirit and those of our ancestors, and as a Christian, I couldn't." He first had to bury his father.

There is nothing foreign or out-of-date about the stories Jesus told the crowds who followed him—not for the people of Korea. And Jesus—who mixed with common folk, who was familiar with their lives, who himself had no home, who was followed by crowds, who taught them and healed their diseases—is one they can understand, love, and follow to the death as many did in the communist war in Korea.

-16-

Dr. Koh and I consulted together frequently and assisted one another with difficult operations, he in general surgery, I in obstetrical and gynecological work. In the outpatient dispensary our examining rooms were on either side of the treatment room. If one of us encountered an unusual or especially interesting condition, we asked the other to see it. There were many fascinating medical and surgical problems not described in any of my medical textbooks.

Liver abscess was a common complication of amoebic dysentery. In Canada, I'd never seen such an abscess. Since textbooks said the only treatment was surgical, I operated on the first case I had to treat. The patient was a fifteen-year-old boy with a huge tender mass in his upper abdomen. So much liver substance had been destroyed by the abscess that through the incision my finger could not reach any liver tissue at all. There seemed to be nothing but a large cavity full of pus. More than a pint was evacuated and the wound continued to drain for days. No matter how often the dressings were changed the unfortunate lad and his bed were always wet.

Soon after this experience, at a meeting of the Korea Medical Missionary Society, Dr. Alfred I. Ludlow of Severance

Hospital described a new method of treatment he had tried and found successful for liver abscess. Instead of opening the abdomen to evacuate the abscess, he aspirated the pus through a hollow needle and injected through the needle directly into the abscess cavity a dose of the remedy found most useful in the treatment of amoebic dysentery. The medicine could also be given by mouth. There was no painful wound, no mess for the nurses to clean up; the patients were more comfortable and recovered in a shorter time. I never drained a liver abscess again. Dr. Ludlow's treatment was a great advance.

Dr. Ludlow was not the only missionary doctor to contribute to medical knowledge. *The China Medical Journal,* published in China in an English edition with articles by various missionary doctors, was the best source of information on the tropical diseases found in South East Asia. It gave methods of diagnosis and treatment worked out in mission hospitals that hadn't found their way into any standard textbook.

A disease then prevalent among foreigners in the Orient, and thought to be uncommon among Orientals, was sprue. The cause was unknown and the treatment was a matter of trying anything you could think of. No known treatment was satisfactory and many Westerners left the country for a change of diet and climate, while not a few became permanent invalids. Fortunately, there is now an adequate treatment and sprue will never again be the scourge it was.

In spite of the prevalance of parasites and acute infectious diseases, life in Korea had compensating circumstances. In the bull-cart age, there were practically no traffic accidents and if one did occur it was seldom serious. Bicycles were the chief safety hazards.

A boy who fell off his bicycle over the end of a bridge sustained a fractured arm. An hour after Dr. Koh had reduced the fracture and put the arm in a plaster cast, I went to see how the boy was feeling. He was so pale I feared he must have other injuries. Further examination revealed a ruptured spleen. The anemia was due to internal hemorrhage. Immediate operation was required to remove the badly damaged organ and stop the bleeding. Blood transfusion would normally be given in such cases now, but even though blood was not available, he made a good recovery.

The most frequent cause of internal hemorrhage was rupture of the fallopian tube between the uterus and ovary when pregnancy occurred in the tube. The distended organ soon ruptured and severe bleeding resulted. If the operation were delayed, the patient was likely to die from loss of blood. These patients sometimes come with an abdomen full of blood and in such serious condition that the shock of being given a general anesthetic and having a major operation would be more than they could endure.

A request for some of the relatives to give blood for a transfusion resulted in a shrug of the shoulders and the remark that it would be better for the sick person to die than for someone else.

Using a small amount of local anesthetic, I made a short incision in the abdominal wall, removed some of the patient's own blood from the abdominal cavity, and transfused it back into her veins. This resulted in sufficient improvement in pulse and blood pressure to make it reasonably safe to give an anesthetic and remove the bleeding tube. When the source of bleeding was removed, the patient's condition responded to the usual methods of treatment. All of many such cases recovered except one who was in a dying condition on arrival and succumbed before anything could be done.

Large tumors were frequent. Abdominal cysts that could fill a big bucket when removed were all in the day's work. If not previously treated by the *chim,* they were generally quite easily removed. If they had been punctured many times, the resulting adhesions made surgery difficult and time consuming. One tiny young woman had in addition to an enormous ovarian cyst an eight-month pregnancy. She could hardly stagger under the combined weight, and her heart and lungs were so compressed she could scarcely breathe. An operation was risky, but she couldn't survive long as she was. I removed the cyst with difficulty and a few days later, the woman went home, in comfort and very happy. The pregnancy, which in cases of extensive surgery is likely to terminate early, was unaffected.

A woman walked into the clinic one day, her head dragged over to one side by the weight of a tumor bigger than her head. She supported the mass with one hand, while she supported her elbow with her other hand. The tumor was of the parotid gland in front of and under the ear—the gland most often involved in mumps. Over the years, the weight of the growth had pulled it out from between the muscles, vessels, and nerves that normally surround the parotid. It was now suspended by a sort of broad stalk; I thought I could remove it without too much difficulty or danger. My fingers were itching to get at it, but the woman was so attached to it after carrying it about for thirty years that she couldn't bear to part with it, and I lost the opportunity to acquire an interesting specimen. I took some good photographs but lost them along with all my notes, records, and pictures when we were exchanged for the Japanese interned in Canada and the United States during World War II.

Another interesting case was that of a woman with three separate tumors in her lower abdomen. One was surprisingly hard. I diagnosed uterine fibroids, one of which had become calcified. The others were getting larger and causing trouble. At operation I found a real pathological collection. She had a fibroid tumor, an ovarian cyst, and a calcified fetus or "stone baby." A calcified fetus is the result of a pregnancy outside the uterus in the abdominal cavity. As there is no way for it to be born, it dies, and, over the years, shrinks and becomes calcified till it is stony hard.

On asking the woman about it later, she told of a pregnancy fourteen years previously that she had considered normal till the time came for delivery. She had a few pains, but the baby never was born. In the next few months her abdomen slowly decreased in size except for a lump that gradually became harder and harder. As it never caused any pain, she didn't bother to see a doctor about it. Only recently, when two other lumps appeared and were getting larger, did she go to a doctor for an examination. It never occurred to her to mention the former pregnancy with its unusual result.

Patients generally were willing to leave tumors behind and we acquired them for our collection of pathological specimens used in teaching. Amputated limbs were another matter. They were a natural part of the body and must be buried in the same grave as the original owner so that he would have a complete body in the spirit world. They were taken home and buried in an auspicious place to await the arrival of the rest of the body, whenever that might be.

Although traffic accidents were rare, those in homes and factories were not. Among the commonest were burns and scalds. Children fell into burning braziers, or their clothes caught fire from going too close to them, or they pulled pots of boiling soup onto themselves. Such injuries were commonly treated at home by applying road dust, cobwebs, or fecal matter under a covering with cabbage leaves. Burns were invariably infected when we first saw them, which made it useless to do skin grafts at an early stage. The result was delayed healing with much scarring, often followed by contraction, not only of the skin, but the tissues underneath. Usually it was on account of the disfiguring or handicapping complications that the patient, months after the injury, first went to a doctor.

Worse than the usual burns and scalds of the skin were burns of the mouth, gullet, and stomach from drinking a solution of washing soda or lye. This was either accidental or for the purpose of suicide. As washing soda was used for whitening clothes and every household had some on hand, children often got hold of it thinking it was water and took a mouthful.

A distraught man once brought his fourteen-year-old son who had drunk lye after his father told him he couldn't afford to send him to high school. The disappointment was more than the boy could take. About two hours after he drank the lye the pair arrived at the hospital. The agony of the unfortunate lad was distressing to see. Lips, mouth, throat, and no doubt the gullet and lining of the stomach were burned white. Though unable to speak, the boy made us understand he wanted water to cool the burning sensation, but he was quite unable to swallow it. He struggled to tell us he wanted to live. The distress of the father was almost as great as that of the son. He pleaded with us to save his boy and blamed himself for the tragic affair. We did what we could to relieve the lad's suffering, but he died within an hour of arrival at the hospital.

Another young man wishing to commit suicide chewed a lump of dry lye, but was unable to swallow it. Though his mouth was badly burned, his stomach escaped injury. He survived without the serious consequences that followed damage to the esophagus and stomach.

Such patients, if they survived the early acute effects, were usually able to take fluids and soft foods for a few weeks. Then scar tissue that formed following the injury began to contract. The esophagus often became so narrowed that swallowing was difficult or impossible. Some of these people arrived at the hospital only after several days of starvation.

Occasionally it was possible to dilate the constriction, but more often an operation was needed to place a tube in the stomach through the abdominal wall to permit feeding while dilation was being carried out, or to get the patient well nourished enough to withstand a major operation. Some refused to have a second operation, though life with a tube was far from enviable and more than once such patient declared she would rather be dead, for most of these unfortunates were women. Without modern anesthesia and blood transfusions, the extensive surgery now possible to provide a new esophagus was not then practicable.

Sometimes our best efforts were in vain.

Elder Han brought one of his sons to the hospital after several months illness from kidney disease. The seventeen-year-old boy was pale and weak, his body considerably swollen with the fluid his inflamed kidneys were unable to excrete. Since his condition was obviously serious and deteriorating, the family at last brought him to Cheihei Hospital. We gave him the best treatment then available, including a strictly limited diet to ease the work of the kidneys. On this regimen, he made slow but continuous improvement. When the swelling had all disappeared, the boy thought he was cured and wanted to go home.

When his mother came asking me to discharge him, I explained the serious nature of his illness, its long duration, and pointed out the improvement with treatment. I told her that unless the diet was continued for a considerable time, the trouble would soon recur, and a second recovery could not be expected. She agreed to let him stay.

Half an hour later, the father announced he was taking his son home. I repeated what I told the mother, but the elder was determined to let the boy have his way.

"Why?," I asked, "when he's doing so well, why must you take him home now? If he leaves now and returns to his former diet, he'll soon be as sick as before."

"He's crying to go home," said the father, "so what can I do?"

"You may as well buy a coffin then," I said, "for you'll soon need it." This was cruel, but I hoped to shock the man into a realization of the situation.

They went.

Three days later an elder brother brought the patient back unconscious and more swollen than before.

"What happened?" I asked.

"My younger brother was starved for so long in the hospital he wanted to eat everything, so Mother cooked all the things he liked best and gave a big feast. He ate as much as he could and father called in all the doctors he could get in touch with and got medicine from each of them. My brother took all of it, so why he should have got like this we can't understand."

That afternoon they bought the coffin and took the body home in it.

Typhoid fever occurred sporadically all the year around but was prevalent every summer. There were frequent serious complications and, at that time, no specific treatment. Typhus was less frequent, and although Koreans got milder cases, it was usually fatal in foreigners. The first effective innoculation against typhus was developed by a missionary in China whose mission had been decimated by it, but that came later. Two girls admitted with typhus did not feel very ill and sat up in bed demanding a full diet for each meal even when their temperature reached forty degrees centigrade or one hundred four fahrenheit.

This was the disease that had carried off Dr. MacMillan. When Ada Sandell developed it, she went as near death's door as anyone I ever saw who returned from it. I was watching her one night when she was so weak I couldn't get her pulse or be sure she was breathing. She seemed quite unconscious and I couldn't determine if she was still alive. As I bent over her, watching closely, praying, and feeling for her pulse, her right upper eyelid quivered. That was the first sign of life in an hour. In a few minutes the eyelid quivered again, and a little later the left one quivered as well. Then one eye partly opened and soon after I could see that she was breathing feebly. A little later I was able to detect the pulse. It was days before she could speak or lift a hand, and it took months to get her strength back.

Because of the large number of tuberculosis victims, the limited accommodations available for them, and the ignorance of the disease, it was the greatest public health problem. We fitted up the basement of our small tuberculosis annex to take ten more patients. This made thirty beds for such patients, and that was the total number in the province. The basement didn't get much direct sunlight, but was airy and brightly painted. Patients there seemed to do as well as those on the upper floor.

Our x-ray equipment would not be permitted in any institution today because the operator was not protected from the radiation the exposed bare power lines emitted. Such a machine was the only one the hospital could afford. It was the last of its type, for the very next year better models with enclosed wires and adequate insulation were available. I ran it myself until I taught one of our graduate nurses to take x-ray pictures and later trained a full-time technician.

A leaded rubber apron and gloves gave me reasonable protection and I kept as far away as possible from the source of the rays. The problem was to keep others away. No patient would enter the room without the presence of some of his family. Since he himself had to be in the proper place and position for the exposure to be made, he was safe enough. Others were not so easily controlled. They wanted to see all that was to be seen and, in spite of warnings to keep away from the apparatus, especially the exposed wires at the back, they were inclined to wander over there. Fortunately no one ever sustained a burn or electric shock, and the negatives produced by that little machine, within its limitations, were quite satisfactory. Of course, it couldn't do all that a more powerful unit would, but it showed bones and chests quite well. With so much active tuberculosis and so many suspected cases, chest films were the most frequent of all.

Some people had strange ideas about x-rays. While I was getting the equipment ready, one young man broke into sobs.

"What's the matter?" I asked. "Surely you're not having that much pain."

"Ma je mak!" "This is the end!" he said. He expected to die. He was convinced that when an x-ray examination was advised, he hadn't long to live. Attempts to reassure him were not very successful at the time, but later, when he realized he was getting better, he forgot his fears.

Every patient and his family had to see the film for themselves. Some expected to recognize themselves as in a regular photograph. One man complained loudly that his film was spoiled and demanded his money back.

"Spoiled! What do you mean?" I asked. "This is a good clear film that shows what we needed to see to help diagnose your trouble."

"Look at all those curved lines on it. How can you say it's

not spoiled? There are no lines like that on me."

"Of course there are no lines like that on the outside of you, but this x-ray picture shows the inside. We don't need a picture of the outside. We can see that for ourselves, but we want to know if there's any disease in your lungs. Those lines are the shadows of your ribs, and the lungs showing between the ribs look quite healthy. If we couldn't see the shadows of the ribs, we couldn't see the lungs either."

This explanation mollified him somewhat.

Most wanted to take the film home to show their friends. I explained that what they paid for was not the film, but the use of the machine and the knowledge and skill of the doctor in diagnosing the condition. They were rarely satisfied with that explanation and sometimes became abusive unless given the film. Though I told them it would be needed later to compare with the next x-ray picture to be taken to see what progress was being made, they seldom brought it back. If they did, it was usually so soiled and battered that proper comparison was impossible.

One film I particularly regretted losing in this way was the abdomen of a man complaining of stomach pain. I wanted to see if an ulcer were present. To my amazement, the negative showed thirteen nails in various parts of the abdomen, three of them embedded in the spine where one had been driven in with such force it had broken off.

"How in the world did you get all these nails in your abdomen?" I inquired.

"Oh, that," was the reply. "I never thought to mention that. It happened fourteen years ago. I had the same trouble then and went to a doctor who drove the nails in to cure the pain."

"What kind of nails were they? They don't seem to have rusted or caused you any special distress."

"They couldn't rust. They were copper nails."

"Were you better after that treatment?"

"I thought I was better for a while, but the pain soon came back."

"Didn't the pain sometimes get better for a while and come back again other times too?"

"Sometimes I'd be almost free of pain for a few weeks, but it always came back. Now that I've had the x-ray I'll be cured, won't I?"

"The x-ray picture is to show whether you have an ulcer that can be cured by an operation, and if so, just where the ulcer is. The x-ray picture won't cure you, but it shows an ulcer, and if you want us to operate, I think we can help you."

"Give me the picture."

I hoped to show these remarkable films to some of my medical friends in Canada and did my best to retain them. The man demanded the films and when his manner grew threatening I compromised and we each took one. He went off with his and I never saw him again.

A few of our tuberculosis patients were equally lacking in understanding and cooperation.

Among the first patients to be admitted to our tuberculosis wards was a young woman, Pak Jin-Ju, who had had some training as a nurse under Dr. MacMillan. A slight hemorrhage from the lung alerted her to her condition and she came to the hospital in deep despair. She was a young widow with two children to support and no hope of being able to do it. She turned her face to the wall, refused to eat, or even to talk to visiting friends, or to me. Her one reply to my cheerful morning greetings was, "I'm going to die. I know I am."

"We're all going to die sometime," I replied, "but it needn't be soon for you. You've every chance of getting better if you do what I tell you."

"No. I'm going to die. Nothing's any use."

"It's foolish to talk like that. Many people much sicker than you have recovered. But you must eat. How can anyone be strong who refuses to eat? No one else can do that for you."

"Who'll look after my fatherless children and my old mother when I'm gone?"

"You will if you do your part to get well."

"I know I'm going to die," and she turned her face to the wall.

Another young woman from the Changjin Mountains where there were no doctors arrived at the hospital at about the same time as Jin-Ju.

Hoping she might get better without treatment, her family waited for months before bringing her. Now she was in a sad state. Not only were her lungs grossly diseased, but her digestive tract as well. She was unable to eat much and retained little of that. She had high fever, severe pain, and constant cough that disturbed her rest. Though her condition appeared hopeless, she was much too sick to stand the fifty-mile trip by bull cart back to her home, and we admitted her.

Now that she was in hospital, she was confident she would be cured. It was too late for that, but she was cheerful and cooperative and we did our best for her. She responded to the treatment of her symptoms and, before long, her pain was relieved and she was able to retain nourishment. She gained strength and improved more than we had dared to hope for. After a few months, she returned home.

Jin-Ju too went home in six months, still in a despondent mood, and considerably worse than on admission. The contrast between the two patients was remarkable. The seemingly hopeless one, who had confidence, improved, while the other with only a slight disease, who was depressed and noncooperative, lost ground.

By the time Jin-Ju left the hospital, her sister had developed the disease. Jin-Ju, afraid of infecting her children, had her mother build a little shack in the courtyard where she had a bed made of planks. The old mother looked after her two sick daughters and the children all through the cold winter. She took Jin-Ju's meals to her in the shack, though the sick woman still refused to eat much. The mother attended to all her daughter's needs, though when she first went home she was able to attend to them herself.

Though she seldom paid attention to my advice, she sent for me often. Friends found her so discouraged and difficult that they stopped coming to see her.

The old mother had known hard times before. Her husband had abandoned his family when the daughters were small. What use was a wife who failed to produce a son? The mother had to earn the living as well as bring up her children. The husband was said to have consoled himself with no less than seven concubines.

One of the first problems I heard discussed in the mission station after arriving in Hamheung was how to help this family. The mother worked in one of the mission houses, saved her money, and built a small house nearby. It was registered in her name. The husband, evidently needing money for his entourage, put the house up for sale. Women had few rights in Korea, and a husband could do as he liked with his wife's property.

There was nothing in the mission budget for such a contingency. What could be done? I had brought a few hundred dollars with me for hospital equipment. This seemed more urgent. I bought the house, and Nu-Dia and her family continued to live in it.

Loud screams from their yard one day brought Mr. Scott running from his house higher up the hill to see what was the matter. One of the husband's concubines had come demanding dishes for her establishment. Nu-Dia who bought her belongings by her own labor was disinclined to give them up to one of her supplanters. She refused, and the young woman began to beat the older one. Jin-Ju, watching helpless from her bed in the doorless shack, added her screams, with what breath she had, to her mother's.

"What's going on here?" demanded Mr. Scott shocked at what he saw. The concubine finding herself in the minority left without the dishes.

After leaving the hospital, Jin-Ju never rose from her bed. She gradually became weaker, more depressed, and more demanding. Every time she had a headache or a new worry came to mind she sent for me. There wasn't much I could do but try to allay some of the most distressing symptoms and provide some light nourishment. If she didn't eat it, one of the others would.

For months, she lay on her bed of planks, a thick quilt underneath and another over her. She gradually became weaker till she was no longer able to turn over or straighten her limbs. At last, a message from her mother came once more. "Jin-Ju's dying. Please come this last time." When the labored breathing stopped, I put the worn and weary old mother gently to bed on the warm floor in her house. She weighed little more than the daughter who had just died.

The condition of another tuberculosis victim was so distressing he could hardly be turned away even though there was no hope of a cure. However, with rest, good food, and treatment of his troublesome symptoms, these subsided, and he made considerable temporary improvement.

Every evening, Elder Lee had prayers in the corridor of the little tuberculosis hospital. Most patients enjoyed the singing and wished to listen to the brief service, but the new man asked that his door be closed. Even with the door closed, he heard the singing, decided he liked the music, and asked to have the door open during the singing. When he heard the words as well as the tune he found they weren't at all what he expected. This didn't sound like superstition. In a short time he asked to have the door open for the whole devotional period. He decided he couldn't object to anything said, and much of it was good. Everybody knew there were spirits. Why shouldn't there be a Great Spirit God? He wanted to hear more, and when the elder bade him good night, he had questions to ask.

"To love your enemies," he said, "that is truly wonderful, but how can it be done? I want to know more about this. Can you get me a Book for myself?"

He got his New Testament, read it, in intervals of coughing, and asked more questions. "Why did this Jesus, who had power to heal and to still the waves, let himself be killed?"

"Because he loved men, and saw that nothing less than his death would make them realize how evil they were. He was willing to suffer pain, shame, and death for that."

"I believe this in spite of myself," the young man said. "I

can't help it. I want to be a follower of that man Jesus. How do I start?"

"Just tell him you're sorry for your past ingratitude and neglect of his love and mercy, and ask him to forgive you and accept you as his child."

"But I'm a communist," he whispered, "and have said all sorts of bad things about God, the church, and Christians. I didn't even want to come to this Christian hospital, but no one else would do anything for me."

"Jesus is waiting to forgive you as soon as you turn to him."

A spell of coughing interrupted the conversation. When the sick man could speak again, he closed his sunken eyes and prayed. "Jesus, I didn't know about you and how good you are. Now that I know, I'm sorry I hated you and your followers and said evil things about you. Please forgive me in spite of how bad I've been. I'm sorry I haven't much time left to show you I love you because you loved me even while I hated you."

"Amen," said Lee Changno. "Loving and merciful God, thank you for forgiving and accepting this brother who's been straying alone for a long time. He is sick and in distress but has come to you now. Bless him, comfort him, and guide him each day till you call him home to be with you for ever. Amen."

A happy face greeted me next morning when the young communist told me he was now a Christian.

A few months later, after recovering as much as was possible considering his badly damaged lungs, he left the hospital and went to his father's house. His father met him at the gate.

"I hear you've joined the Jesus fanatics," he said. "Is that so?"

"Yes, Father, I'm now a follower of Jesus."

"Then you can't come in here. There'll be none of those rascals in my house. Go away."

"Father, where can I go?"

"Anywhere you like. I'm not having any Jesus people here."

"Then, Father, remain in peace."

When he had become unable to work, his wife had gone back to her parents. He went to see her now, and her family, though not Christians, took him in.

Each fine day he hobbled with his stick to the roadside and sat in the sun. Passing friends stopped to ask how he was.

"I'm happy," he said. "This sickness has turned out to be a blessing."

"A blessing! How can you say that?"

"If I hadn't been sick, I wouldn't have gone to the hospital where I learned about Jesus. Now, though, I can't expect to get better, my mind is at peace, such peace as I never knew before, and I've no more fear of death. Isn't that a blessing?"

Strange indeed, mused the friends. He's really happy in spite of being sick, turned out of his father's house, in poverty, and distressed by those awful coughing spells. There must be something in this Jesus business.

There by the roadside he taught them what he could, and one day when Elder Lee visited him he learned that eight of his friends had decided to become Christians.

"Please, Elder Lee," said the sick man, "come and teach them how to pray and worship and start a church. There's no church in this district, and they need to know more of what it means to be a Christian."

The elder taught them. As the young man who was such a new Christian himself grew weaker, he had the joy of seeing the little group he had led to his Master grow stronger. He was happy to know that in the short time left to him on earth he had been able to do something for his Master. He had not lived in vain.

-17-

"Pouine," said Kang Do-Ka gently, "my daughter-in-law isn't well at all and she's having another baby. I must leave the hospital and go and help her."

Do-Ka was well past the age when a Korean woman was expected to work. Everybody now called her grandmother.

"But you're not strong enough to do heavy work," I protested. "Isn't there someone else who can help her? How old is your oldest granddaughter?"

"She's sixteen, but she should graduate from middle school this year and nothing can interfere with that. I must go. It's time for me to stop work here anyway. Remember, I'm over sixty now."

She wrapped up her few possessions in a square of cloth tied neatly by the corners, her bedding in another, and was ready. I drove her to the village where her son and his family lived.

On Sunday mornings one member of the hospital evangelistic team stopped off at her village to teach in the little Sunday school and preach at the worship service held at her house. I used to stop and see her when I picked up the team on the way back from the other villages where they taught Sunday school and helped the churches.

One day she told me her plans for her burial.

"*Pouine,* come outside. I want to show you something. That hilltop up there is the place I want to be buried. It's quiet and I often go there to pray. I like to watch the sun go down behind the mountains beyond the plain. It makes me think of the gates of heaven."

"Yes, that's a beautiful spot, but who owns the land? Are you sure there won't be any problem?"

"I've bought a piece of land up there large enough for a gravesite, and told my son about it, so it's all settled. Now, let's go in and see the grave clothes I've made. I want to be buried respectably as all my family have been."

Opening a drawer in the lacquered wardrobe in her room, she took out an outfit of handwoven white silk. She showed me a pair of the long loose trousers women wore under their wide pleated skirts, a skirt to match, and the short jacket with long ties to go with it. She handed the clothing to me.

"I want to be buried in these things," she said. "Now everything is ready."

"These garments are lovely," I said, fingering the soft, white silk and admiring the tiny, hand-sewn stitches. When the day comes that these are needed, there will be many lonely people in this community, I thought, and I'll be one of them.

"My daughter-in-law and my grandchildren are all so good to me that if only my son were a Christian I'd be very happy. As you know, he doesn't come to worship, but he doesn't object to our having the Sunday school and worship here. He doesn't work much and my pension doesn't go far in this household, but I thank God for my daughter-in-law and the children."

Some weeks later, Elder Lee, concern in his voice, told me, "Grandmother Kang's in deep trouble."

"What's the matter?"

"Her useless son's got in debt and is advertising her house for sale. If it's sold, they'll all be turned out, and where can the poor old woman go?"

"But isn't it *her* house, registered in her name? I remember when she bought it, for I lent her money to help buy it. How can he sell it?"

"Isn't he a man? What can an old woman do?"

"Who'll buy a house if they can't get the title to it?"

"Anyone who wants the house and can pay for it will pass a gift to the police and they'll fix it up."

"Then what can be done? Is anyone bargaining for the house or is there still a chance for us to do something about it?"

The elder said he would find out. He reported next day the house had not been sold. I bought it for fifty dollars, a fair price for such a village house in those days, and had it registered in my name so Do-Ka would have a roof over her head as long as she needed it. Neither of us mentioned it, and I hope she never knew of her son's intentions.

While Grandmother Kang's house was thus preserved for her, other friends met with tragedy.

Edna McLellan, on returning from a month's teaching in the mountains, told us of the sorrow that came to the village where Elder Kim and his middle-aged wife Wha-Soon, who married at the age of forty-three, were living. Their precious little son was now nearly a year old, the pride and joy of the household.

"While I was there," said Edna, "some of the small children of the village took sick, but nobody paid much attention. Children were often sick and generally got better in a few days. Anyway, there was no doctor to take them to. When, after a couple of days of crying, the sick children began to have convulsions and became so sleepy they couldn't be roused, the parents became alarmed. Nobody knew what to do. Some called in the *mudang* and, though she did her best, every sick child died.

"When Elder Kim's son took ill, the family were nearly frantic. They now knew this was a serious disease needing more expert care than was available. It would take four days to reach the hospital in Hamheung and the other children had died after four or five days illness. They could never reach the hospital in time.

"The Christians came to comfort the parents and pray for the child. Non-Christian neighbors urged them to try the *mudang,* but they had no faith in the sorceress, nor did it agree with their Christian beliefs to use her and her relations with evil spirits. The neighbors insisted that if they let their child die without having the *mudang* everyone would blame them for the death.

"The parents had little faith in the old style practitioner of herb medicine, but were desperate enough to try almost anything. They sent for him. By the time he arrived, the little lad was unconscious so I hope he didn't feel the red-hot needles the man thrust into each tiny finger and toe. The doctor then collected his fee and departed, saying he had done all he could. In half an hour the baby died." Edna's voice shook, and she wiped away a tear.

"The elder prayed that God would comfort his wife. Wha-Soon and some of the neighbors began the wailing for the dead. '*Aigo. Aigo.*' The mother beat her breast and pounded her fists against the wall in grief and despair. I don't think she slept at all until after the funeral on the third day, when she was utterly exhausted."

"The poor parents," said Ada. "That was a hard experience for anyone, but for them, knowing that at their age they'll not have another child, it was unusually bitter."

"Has Wha-Soon become at all reconciled to her loss?" I asked.

"That's the saddest part of it," Edna replied, walking up and down as she talked. "She blamed herself for what happened. If only she had realized at once how serious the illness was and started for the hospital then; if only she'd taken better care of the child; if only she'd done differently; if only . . . if only. . . . It was all her fault. How could her husband now endure the sight of her when he knows her to be the cause of the loss of his son? Between grief and self-blame she was quite distraught."

"What did the elder say to that?" I asked.

"He tried to comfort her and so did the neighbors and especially the church people, but she couldn't forgive herself and felt sure everybody must be secretly blaming her. Elder Kim really was wonderful. I did my best too, but she wouldn't listen to anyone." Edna dropped into a chair and clasped her hands.

"Three days after the funeral, Wha-Soon left home, saying that since she knew her husband couldn't bear the sight of her, she was going to Wonsan to get a job in a church there."

She worked in one of the Wonsan churches to the satisfaction of the people till time began to blunt the edge of her grief. More than a year later, she heard that her husband had developed painful arthritis and was becoming quite crippled. She then realized she had selfishly run away from her duty. So the lonely man got his wife back, she nursed him tenderly, and they comforted one another.

Missionaries too had their misfortunes.

A few days after Jennie Robb went to teach for a month at a rural Bible institute near the Siberian border, a messenger boy ran into our hospital. Shouting *"Chunbo! Chunbo!"* ("telegram"), he tossed a yellow sheet in my door and dashed off. The telegram was from Dr. Whang, a young man recently graduated from Severance Medical College who had set up practice in the far north. Miss Robb was in his hospital with a fractured leg. Would I please come and get her.

I took the next train north. It was the dead of winter, bitter cold, and there was much snow in the mountains. I had to change trains in the night at a junction and get a slow local to Heisanjin where Dr. Whang met me. His grandfather was one of the first Christians in the Wonsan district. When Miss Robb traveled there, she frequently stayed at their house and knew all the family including this young doctor who thought of her almost as his own grandmother.

The previous evening after finishing her teaching, while walking back to Dr. Whang's house where she was staying, she slipped on a snow-covered patch of ice. She came down heavily on the frozen road and felt a bone snap in her leg. Unable to rise and suffering severe pain, she would soon be frostbitten if not rescued quickly. Though she called to passersby, they were unconcerned and went their way.

She was getting very cold when at last one stopped and she asked him to send word of her accident to Dr. Whang. In a short time the doctor arrived with splints, bandages, a stretcher, and a man to help carry her.

In his small private hospital with four or five beds, Dr. Whang made her as comfortable as possible. He reduced the fracture and splinted the limb with the bones in good position.

It didn't seem wise to undertake a long journey including a change of trains with nothing but splints to control the fracture, so the doctor and I put on a plaster cast. We waited till it dried before starting because a wet cast might not retain its shape and in zero weather might freeze. It seemed almost cold enough in the hospital room for it to freeze.

I had a bed next to Miss Robb. The family lived in hot floor rooms and, when I was not with Jennie or in bed, I stayed with them. To get there meant thrusting feet into slippers as cold and stiff as ice and walking on the outside veranda from one end of the house to the other. The Whang family didn't seem to mind the cold. They did their best for us by providing extra quilts and cooking special food. We couldn't impose on their kindness longer than necessary. Jennie was anxious to get home, and there was work waiting for me in the hospital. I sent a telegram to the little church at the railway junction where we had to change trains to ask that somebody meet the midnight train and help carry Miss Robb to the southbound express.

About twenty of the church people were there, with a homemade stretcher on which they carried her gently to the other train. What a wonderful thing is this fellowship of Christians that we could confidently appeal to people we never met and a whole church would turn out on a bitterly cold midnight to help.

At Hamheung next morning, hospital orderlies met the train with a stretcher. An x-ray examination showed the bones in good position. We took Jennie home to our house where under my supervision and with Ada's nursing she made good progress and was soon planning for another country trip.

Not all missionary illness had as happy an ending.

A telegram from Dr. Demares of the Methodist Mission at Wonsan brought me on the next train to see Reverend D. A. Macdonald, one of our United Church missionaries. He had taken sick the previous day while he and his wife were packing up at Wonsan Beach to return home after their summer holiday. He felt wretched and thought he was getting another attack of malaria, but they set out. Their house was on top of a high hill in Wonsan city. Halfway up was the home of the women missionaries, Elizabeth and Louise McCully. The road was steep and they had to walk up. Mr. Macdonald managed to reach the women's house, but could go no farther. They sent for Dr. Demares who saw that his condition was serious and wired for me, the doctor responsible for the health of our mission members. I caught the next train and when I arrived Mr. Macdonald was unconscious.

Within the past few days Dr. Demares had seen several similar cases all of whom had died. There was no hope for our colleague. These were the first cases in an epidemic of encephalitis, the inflammation of the brain commonly known as sleeping sickness. Mr. Macdonald died that night. When I got back to Hamheung, I found three such patients in our hospital.

The Macdonald sons were at college in Canada and Mrs. Macdonald was alone. Korean and mission friends rallied around to comfort her and she amazed everyone by her quiet courage. Long before this illness, her husband had said he wished, when the time came, to be cremated. His wife requested that this wish be carried out.

A memorial service in Wonsan was attended by a great crowd of friends, both Korean and foreign. The body was then brought to Hamheung where a funeral service was held on the grounds of Yungsaing Girls' School since those who wished to attend were more than could be accommodated in any of the churches. Hymns of praise, comfort, and triumph and words of hope, together with the absence of wailing, made a contrast to the burial practices of non-Christians. "For neither life nor death . . . nor anything else in God's whole world has any power to separate us from the love of God in Christ our Lord."

And so our friend who had endeared himself to all by his kindliness and good humor left us. Perhaps it is for his sense of fun and his role as a peacemaker that we remember him best.

-18-

The Great Depression that settled over the Western world soon affected us in Korea and in other mission areas. As church contributions in Canada decreased during the hard times, the mission board advised us not to ask for any increase in funds to provide for the increasing work. Then came cuts in our estimated budget. In order to use church money to the best advantage and make it go as far as possible, the mission had always practiced economy. In the financial emergency, missionaries asked that, rather than cut the budget for maintenance of the work, their salaries be reduced. This helped for a while, but as the Depression continued and funds were further reduced, the great problem was where to cut down with the least damage to the work.

Finally, when still further curtailment became necessary, the board informed the mission that since their salaries could not be continued, four families would have to retire and return to Canada to find other positions. The board asked the mission to decide which among their number would be retired. A more difficult and distressing decision would be difficult to imagine.

Koreans found it hard to realize there could be any shortage of money in a wealthy Western country, and explanations were not easy. Why was the mission cutting down on subsidies to weak churches when they were having such a struggle to pay their pastors a living salary? Why were scholarships to needy students reduced when there were still poor students who couldn't pay their school fees and more churches than before were waiting for their service?

Each year, we hoped that some of the cuts might be restored, but instead there were more. Fortunately, before the reduction in funds began, the church in the two provinces—North and South Hamkyung—had undertaken to increase local support of their churches by ten percent per year. The mission funds thus freed were to be used to help start new churches.

While the government was demanding larger budgets for mission schools, the grants for schools decreased to the extent that some had to be closed in order that others might continue.

A diversion in these gloomy times was a visit of a Korean prince to his ancestral home near Hamheung. As a child, the prince had been torn away from his native land by the Japanese and had grown up in exile in Japan. He was married to a high-born Japanese lady and now was permitted to return for a first visit to Korea after many years.

Streets were cleaned, garbage removed, signs repainted, fences rebuilt, unsightly objects removed, and streets repaired. Strict orders were issued that no washing was to be hung on clothes lines or fences, all dogs were to be kept off the streets, and everyone was to wear his best clothes.

The day came. The hospital laundrywoman hung out her wash at daybreak so she could take it in long before the prince's train arrived at eleven o'clock, but, in a few minutes, an angry Japanese policeman demanded the laundry be taken in at once. When he caught sight of a small dog on the street, he raised an alarm and a group of excited policemen, Japanese and Korean, gave chase. By the time they finally cornered the dog, it was far from its home. As it couldn't tell them where it belonged, they were unable to punish the owner.

By half past ten, I realized that all the patients had been attended to, no more were coming to the clinic, and most of the staff had disappeared. I decided I might as well go too when I caught sight of Elder Kim, assistant to Edna McLellan.

"Where's everybody, Kim Changno?" I asked.

"All gone to the station to see the prince."

"Why don't we go too?"

"It's too late now. People were to have been in their assigned places half an hour ago."

"Let's take the car and go see what we can."

Off we went through the deserted streets till we came to the long columns of people lining both sides of the main highway from the station. Policemen were on guard every few yards to keep the crowds well back from where the royal party was to pass. Once between the lines, there was no place to turn off and the police, evidently thinking that anyone coming so boldly at that hour had a right to be there, waved us on.

We went flying past the little group of foreigners stationed as far as possible from the place of honor where the prince was to alight from the train. On seeing us, they were much concerned, fearing we would pay dearly for our foolhardiness. Word had reached them, though it somehow missed getting to me, of our appointed place in the line up.

All eyes were on us and the police continued to wave us on. Elder Kim was thrilled.

"This is glorious!" he exclaimed. "Never did I imagine myself in the public eye."

I was getting worried, but there was nothing to do but go on and hope there would be parking space near the station. The grounds were crowded and we had to go beyond them to find a place to stop. When the prince and his party arrived, we saw no more of him in the crowd than if we had remained in the hospital.

My missionary colleagues reprimanded me for being so reckless. Since the police were too busy seeing that the prince didn't peek into any corner they didn't want him to see and since none of his countrymen were able to approach him, our escapade was overlooked. I wasn't overwhelmed with remorse, and nothing could take Elder Kim's moment of glory away from him.

Since contacts with minor Japanese officials were frequently unpleasant, I contrived to have as few as possible. The hospital had to make reports, and I had to have the car inspected by police regularly.

If we went anywhere by train, we had to tell the policemen at the station where we were going, and why, how long we expected to stay, and where. They also asked one's age, when one had first come to Korea, if one's parents were living, and what one's father's profession was. Any signs of impatience in answering these questions aroused suspicions and resulted in a still more detailed inquiry. All the answers were recorded in a small notebook.

Once through the wicket, another policeman on the platform would ask the same questions and make notes of each reply. On board the train, a third repeated the questions, while the other two compared notes and telephoned the police at the destination to be on the lookout for us. A man in uniform would be awaiting us on the platform with his notebook. Woe betide anyone who, weary of giving the same answers, introduced a little variety.

As soon as one arrived, a policeman would appear where one stayed and demand to see the guest who had to reply to the same questions once more. This was irksome, but it was well to be cooperative.

In those days, each foreigner had a policeman assigned to him whose duty it was to know where the person went, who his friends were, and where he might be found at any particular time. A story went the rounds of one man who kept a diary but forgot to write in it for two or three days and couldn't remember where he was at a certain time. He called up his special policeman and was promptly told.

All our letters were censored and were often delayed at the post office until all interested had time to look them over.

One young woman in Pyengyang, in writing to her mother, mentioned this fact. The very next day a man from the post office came to see her and told her not to worry about her letters being censored because the post office never did such a thing.

Once or twice a year the police inspected the hospital pharmacy. If any bottles of medicine were labeled in English or Korean only, and not also in Japanese, the inspector pronounced the drug unfit for use and smashed the container on the floor. We surmised that he knew nothing whatever about the drugs and wished merely to show his authority and make sure we were using the Japanese language on everything. As neither the man in our pharmacy nor the nursing staff were familiar with all the Japanese names for drugs, we thought it safer to have them labeled with names that we and the staff understood.

Once while I was scrubbing for an operation and anesthetic was being administered to the patient, an urgent message from the office said Japanese officials had come and wanted to see me at once.

"I'm scrubbing for surgery," I replied, "and the patient is already under the anesthetic. I'm sorry, but I can't take them around now. My chief assistant, Dr. Koh, will do the honors. I'm sorry. Ask them to excuse me."

This message was relayed to the officials who were very angry at being shown such disrespect. The messenger reappeared.

"You're to come at once, the officials say. They won't accept any excuse."

So I went at once in my operating cap and mask, soap suds flying from my elbows as I continued to scrub my hands and arms for the regulation time.

Seeing I really was getting ready for an operation and not making an excuse as they had thought, they were overcome with confusion and apologized, saying they would return later. They left and it was months before we saw them again.

On another occasion, the Japanese police brought a dead

body to the hospital and ordered me to do an autopsy. They told me the dead man had committed suicide and I was to state that in my report.

Japanese patients went to the Japanese government hospital. The only ones who ever came to Cheihei Hospital were suffering from venereal disease who wished to keep their condition a secret in government quarters. So I thought it strange that the police should bring this order to me instead of one of their own doctors. Japanese seemed to hate autopsies as much as Koreans, and even in cases where the relatives had given their consent for one, the police, whose permission had also to be obtained, usually refused. It seemed strange that they were now insisting on what they had so often forbidden. They said they would be present and see it done.

The purpose of an autopsy is to discover the cause of death or the nature of the change wrought by the disease in the patient's body. It is therefore quite contrary to all established principles to give instructions beforehand as to what is to be found. I suspected there had been a fight in which the victim was killed and the police wanted to get the killer off by proving suicide.

The autopsy showed seven deep gashes across the front of the neck, the windpipe completely severed, two of the cuts penetrating deeply into the spine. I couldn't imagine any person, no matter how much he might wish to leave this wicked world, making seven such vicious and powerful thrusts into his own neck. I couldn't agree with the police and gave my opinion that the wounds could not have been self-inflicted. On hearing this, they took the body away at once without even thanking me for my trouble. What happened next I don't know, but I suspect another doctor was ordered to do another autopsy and bring in the verdict the police wanted. Why they came to me, I'll never know. Perhaps they thought a woman would be easily intimidated.

One Sunday morning, a wandering beggar without known relatives was found dead in the street near the hospital gate.

In this case, we thought there could be no objection to our doing an autopsy. The unfortunate man had been seen at the hospital some time before and found to be suffering from cancer of the liver. It seemed to be a good and unusual opportunity to study the course of that disease.

We reported the body to the police station at once. They said they were busy, but would send a man around after a while and until he came the body was not to be touched. Hours went by and people began passing on their way to church. With the body lying so near the hospital gate, it looked as though the beggar had been turned away to die. The police didn't come till nearly noon.

When we asked permission to do an autopsy, they not only refused, but said quite unpleasant things about heartless people who would cut up a poor beggar. But because the hospital had tried to help and the body was found at our gate, they insisted that we bury the man.

I once had a different kind of experience with the Japanese.

On the Emperor's birthday, the governor of the province always gave a large celebration party. In addition to officials and military officers, principals of schools and superintendents of hospitals were invited. This included Ethel and me.

After saluting the Japanese flag, bowing to the east, singing the Japanese national anthem, drinking toasts, and listening to congratulatory speeches, guests were invited to partake of refreshments. Tables with various delicacies were scattered here and there about the grounds with an attendant at each to keep the supplies replenished. Each guest had a plate and a pair of chopsticks with which to help himself as he went the rounds of the tables.

I no sooner started with my plate than a drunken Japanese army officer attached himself to me. Everywhere I went, he went too. He took no food for himself but ate whatever I put on my plate. I didn't get a bite. At first it seemed ridiculous, but as he continued to follow me and devour my food; it became annoying. He kept talking to me familiarly in Japanese, which I didn't understand. I could hardly make a scene at the governor's party; everyone else was so intent on enjoying the dainties provided that no one seemed to notice the obnoxious fellow and his bizarre behavior. Finally, when I was at the next to the last table, one of the Japanese ladies observed my plight. Pulling the governor's sleeve, she nodded toward me and my unwelcome companion who, at that moment, placed his face very close to mine. The governor spoke to the official next to him. He, in turn, said a few words in the ear of my satellite who then vanished immediately. By this time, other guests were leaving and there was nothing to do but make my farewells and leave with only one taste of the sumptuous meal that had been prepared.

-19-

Furlough came again in 1935. I left for a year of study and travel among the churches in Canada, while Dr. Koh carried on as acting superintendent in the Cheihei Hospital. Not long after my return to Hamheung the following year, he took a position in Severance Hospital. He had done well and we much regretted his departure.

In his place as surgeon came a big man, strong in body and mind, with a reputation of being hard to get along with. Hamheung was his native place and Mr. McRae had sponsored his study at medical college, which may account for his being willing to come. He had been professor of anatomy at the college and left under more-or-less of a cloud. His knowledge of that subject stood him in good stead, but he had no experience as a surgeon. It wasn't too easy for me to do the surgeon's part of the operation from the assistant's side of the table, while hoping it would appear that he was operating and I assisting. In a short time, he was confident he could handle any surgery by himself and I assisted only in difficult and unusual cases.

In 1937, Japan trumped up the China Incident to provoke war with that country. The isolationist policy of the United States had rendered the League of Nations impotent, the

United Nations Organization hadn't yet come into existence, and other countries didn't want to become involved. After all, China and Japan were on the other side of the world from Europe, and North America had the broad Pacific in between.

While the war spread in China, conditions in Korea became more tense.

Every house and institution was ordered to provide black curtains lined with red for every door and window, and it went hard with any householder who failed to draw them tightly when the blackout alarm went off. Practice blackouts became so frequent that they interfered with all night occupations from student's studying to hospital nursing. During blackouts in the hospital the nurses carried candles in the darkened wards. Police kept sharp watch and soon called at any place showing the least glimmer of light.

One bright moonlight night after the alarm sounded and the hospital was in darkness, the police called up accusing the institution of disobeying orders and having lights on. They demanded that all lights be put out at once. The nurse who took the call was not the subservient type. She answered that every light *was* out. The police said the hospital light could be plainly seen and she would be punished for her reply. She told him that he was seeing the reflection of the moon on the windows and she couldn't put out the moon. If he didn't believe her, he could come and see for himself. He came in haste and had to admit she was right.

Each year more school subjects had to be taught in Japanese. Korean newspapers were severely censored and sometimes appeared with half a page or more blanked out. When a Korean on the Japanese team won the marathon race at the Olympic games one year, there was great jubilation in Korea. The runner, of course, had to appear as a Japanese. When a Korean newspaper printed his picture without the Japanese insignia on his clothing, the newspaper was closed down and the editor imprisoned. Eventually, the Korean papers were ordered to cease publication and schoolchildren were forbidden to speak even a word of their own language on the streets.

A Hamheung boy on his way to school one morning was greeted by a chum from next door who did not go to school. Not knowing Japanese, he of course spoke in Korean. The schoolboy naturally replied in the language he was accustomed to using with his friend and at home with his parents who knew no Japanese.

One of the Japanese teachers, of whom every school had to have a certain number, happened to be coming along behind the boy and heard him speak in Korean. The teacher reported the boy who was promptly expelled from school. This automatically excluded him from any other school, so his education had to stop there. One of the Korean teachers remarked that the punishment seemed a bit severe. For this indiscretion, the teacher was also expelled.

Whatever the circumstances of the case, lawsuits, if between a Korean and a Japanese, were always won by the latter. Under these circumstances, few Koreans even attempted to get their rights through the courts.

In the southern provinces, Koreans had been for years systematically squeezed off their ancestral lands. A certain area would be requisitioned for military purposes. After maneuvers were held, another area would be commandeered, while Japanese farmers settled on the first. The displaced Koreans usually moved to Manchuria or Siberia to get land.

On the plain across the river from Hamheung, the Japanese undertook a large irrigation scheme to increase the production of rice. In the Japanese papers, which none of the farmers could read, there were notices that land was to be expropriated and irrigation canals dug. No one bothered to inform the landowners.

An elderly farmer one morning found a gang of men digging a trench through his land. When he found what they were doing, he went to the local police station to complain that he knew nothing of this and hadn't given his consent. The police gave him a severe beating for his presumption.

When his son heard how his old father had been treated, he went to the police station to object to the beating given his father. As he started to speak, the policeman drew his revolver and shot the son dead.

This caused much indignation in the community, but people were afraid to say anything for fear of reprisals. At the trial, the Japanese policeman who shot the son was sentenced to be transferred to another district.

While laws became more severe and discriminatory, work in the hospital continued to increase. We began to train interns, some of whom stayed on after their training was completed.

One of these was a young woman, Dr. Kim Hyo-Soon, a former graduate of Yungsaing Girls' School where she had led her class. She sang, played the organ, and spoke Japanese so well she was the valedictorian at her graduation. She wanted to study medicine but, at that time, no medical college in Korea was allowed to accept women students. She took medical training at the Tokyo Women's Medical College. Dr. Kim was alert and energetic. Her demure manner was somewhat offset by the twinkle in her bright eyes. She worked with me in obstetrics and gynecology and in the tuberculosis department.

While I was on holiday at Wonsan Beach during the rainy season, there was a great flood in the Hamheung River Valley. We heard at the beach that many houses were washed away and great damage done. Fearing that some of our staff and employees might have lost their homes and be in need of help, I tried to return to the city, but the railroad was washed out in several places and no one knew when traffic would be restored. I then found a small boat bound for Heungnam, the port for Hamheung, and along with many others went aboard. The covered part of the deck was so crowded that one could hardly change position on the straw matting, and anyone who left his place could not find another spot in which to lie down again. I spent the night alternately standing outside in the chill air and trying to squeeze inside the door again to get warm. We entered Heungnam Harbor near daylight. After the usual questions, a policeman ordered a taxi to take me to Hamheung. A Korean boy wanted to go with me and I was going to take him, but the police ordered him away.

At the hospital trouble awaited. Lee Sunsaing blurted out the story.

"Yesterday," he said, "the new surgeon ordered me to pay all the staff salaries because some of our people had damage to their houses from the flood. I told him I had money enough to pay anyone who needed it, but not enough for everybody. Besides, you'd said you would be back in time to arrange for the salaries on the usual date. I told him nobody had asked for his salary, but if anyone needed it, I could pay it.

"With that, he struck me in the face and tore my shirt in sight of all the people in the waiting room. Imagine how shocked I was to be attacked like that! I've never lost so much face in all my life."

"It wasn't your fault," I told him. "You did the right thing and it was unreasonable to blame you. What did you do then?"

"I went into my office and shut the door. What could I do? I didn't want to fight, and he's an older man than I, and much bigger."

"You certainly had a very unpleasant experience, and I think you acted wisely. I'll look into the matter and see what should be done."

"He should leave the hospital," burst out the usually calm and gentle Lee Sunsaing. "He's not a fit person to be on the staff of our Christian hospital."

Inwardly, I agreed with him and wondered uneasily how to handle this situation. In the meantime, there was the damage to employees' homes to be dealt with. Fortunately, it didn't amount to much as most of them lived on higher land nearer the hospital, where the floodwaters failed to reach.

The surgeon's behavior was on my mind all day and I recalled unhappily that he had left Severance after some difficulty with the staff there. I decided to give him time to cool off and reflect on his conduct, hoping his friends might give him good advice in the meantime.

That evening, he came to see me at our house. He said he felt the only thing to do after his unfortunate outburst unbecoming a Christian was to resign. I accepted the resignation gratefully, with what I hope were not too hypocritical words of regret—thankful that the affair was settled with so little trouble. When I heard later that he had gone to the Shinto shrine ceremonies and was urging others of the staff to do the same, I was more thankful he was gone. The authorities were insisting as a patriotic duty that people attend these ceremonies which patriotic Koreans detested and Christians felt were against their conscience. We thought it best not to take up the matter at all, in the hopes that it would be overlooked. If anyone refused to go, he and the institution might be in real trouble.

We had to find another surgeon. The best Severance could do for us was to send a young man who had two years as a surgical resident. He brought his mother, wife, and infant daughter. A slight, pale, young man with delicate features, long, thin fingers, and a shy manner, he looked frail and often said he was sick. Some days he did not come on duty in the afternoon at all. Several times I found he had admitted himself to the hospital during the night and ordered the nurses to give him intravenous injections. He was quite undependable and I began to suspect he might be getting something more than saline in his injections, but apparently he was not.

Meanwhile the financial situation in the West was improving and church contributions increased. Some private donations in addition enabled us to build new brick houses for three of the doctors on the staff. Bricks made in the city penitentiary were the cheapest building material, after mud. Till we had these houses, the doctors had to live anywhere they could rent a suitable house. As none of them had telephones and couldn't be reached at night, I did all the night and emergency work. Everyone was pleased with the fine new houses containing some modern conveniences, and I was grateful to have the doctors on the grounds available for night work and emergencies.

The inpatient wing, the oldest part of the hospital, was showing signs of age. The bricks in the back wall had weathered until only the inside half was left. The foundation had sunk until the floor was uneven. Several of the doors had to be cut off at the bottom to fit the slope of the floors before they could be opened or shut.

Everybody was happy when we were able to demolish and replace the old wing with three stories instead of the former two.

I kept a close watch on the building as it proceeded. If someone didn't, the workmen got careless and the proportion of cement put in concrete work was guessed at instead of measured and was likely to be considerably less than the specifications and contract called for. I had to reject some boards that did not measure up to requirements. The next day, I found them on the third floor about to be slipped into the building without my seeing them. I flung them down and some were so thin and full of knot holes that, on striking the ground, they broke.

An imported enameled bathtub would cost four hundred yen. I found we could build a tile one for fifty. So I measured a regular bathtub the size we wanted, and drew plans of it which gave the measurements and slope.

When the bathtubs were being made, I went out to make sure they conformed to the drawings I'd made. One was being built six feet square filling the whole end of the six-foot wide room. The only way to get to the window would be to go through the bathtub.

"This will never do," I remonstrated. "The bathtub has got to be exactly according to the drawings. Take it down before the cement hardens and make it over."

The workman grumbled, but dismantled the structure. I went back in an hour. This time he was building it four feet square with perfectly vertical walls like the ones in public bath houses where a dozen people bathed together.

"This won't do either," I protested. "It has got to be like the drawings with exactly the same dimensions. Haven't you even looked at the plans I made for it?"

He admitted he hadn't. He said he would lose too much face if he had to dismantle this tub too, so I kicked it to pieces myself. In the end, we had such a nice tub that various others got the plans from me to have similar ones made for themselves. With one completed, there was no difficulty about the others, and we got one on each floor for less than one imported tub would have cost.

We economized in every way we could in order to provide as many facilities as possible. The new part of the building included nurses' stations, utility rooms, toilets and running water, supply cupboards, and a janitor's cupboard for brooms and cleaning materials on each floor. For the first time I had an office to myself. Lee Sunsaing inherited the one we had used together.

The additional floor doubled the bed capacity of the wing from twenty to forty beds, in addition to those over the dispensary.

Soon after we moved into the new wards the young surgeon asked for a holiday by saying he didn't feel well enough to carry on.

"If you're too sick to work you'll have to have a holiday," I told him. "But you haven't been here very long and others work for a year before getting time off. If you're sick, we must find out what the trouble is and see that you get proper treatment. I have to go to Seoul on the night train tonight for a meeting tomorrow, but I'll be back the next night. Can you carry on one more day? You'll be the only surgeon in the hospital."

"All right," he said, "I'll do that. I don't feel any worse than I have for several days. I'll stay on the job till you get back."

A long-distance phone call in Seoul the next day informed me there had been a tragedy and asked me to return at once. I took the night train and arrived next morning.

After talking to me the surgeon went home and lay down on the hot floor. He wouldn't get up to supper or for breakfast the next morning. His mother tried to persuade him to go on duty, but he lay around refusing to eat or talk until the afternoon, when he asked his mother and wife to heat water for a bath. Pleased with this sign of interest in something, his wife placed the three-month-old baby beside him, and the two women filled the Japanese style bathtub with water and lighted a fire underneath. When the water was hot, they went to tell him and found him and the baby lying in a pool of blood. His anatomy textbook was on the low table beside him, open at the page where the large arteries supplying blood to the legs were illustrated. A blood-stained knife lay on the floor beside his body. He had cut both arteries and bled to death.

The mother took this tragedy harder than the wife who had her child to care for. The old mother, long a widow, who worked and saved for years to educate her only son, was left desolate. She thought that he had taken his life to get out of having to support her in her old age. "He's a bad boy," she kept repeating to everyone who came to console her.

I tried in vain to explain that his mind was not normal when he did the reckless deed, and we shouldn't hold him responsible. She wasn't convinced.

When our staff got together to consider the sad event, one after another told of seeing or hearing the unfortunate young man do or say some strange thing. They didn't like to talk about a colleague, and no one person had heard enough to realize his mind was seriously affected. When all the stories were told, it was quite plain he had been in a mental depression that was not recognized.

On questioning the wife and mother, they related still more bizarre behavior that caused them anxiety. Unfortunately, they had kept this to themselves until too late. In retrospect, even if the condition had been diagnosed earlier, I don't know what we could have done. The only psychiatrist in Korea then, as far as I knew, was an Australian, Dr. Charles

McLaren at Severance. It was doubtful if we could have persuaded the young man to go there for treatment, or if there would have been a vacant place for him if he had.

Our next surgeon I found to have had considerably less training and experience than I was led to believe. Once again, I operated from the assistant's side of the operating table while teaching surgery to the supposed surgeon. Fortunately, he was eager to learn and before long could be trusted with ordinary cases while I was there to help with difficulties and complications.

In those busy days, it was good to get away for a little while from the sad stories and sadder sights that so often presented themselves. Grandmother Kang was getting feeble and I tried to go to see her as often as I could. She always appreciated a visit. When she could no longer bow in the graceful Korean way, she would squeeze my hand and give me her gentle smile. After greetings and exchange of news, she would pray for the hospital staff, the patients, for me, and for her wayward son, his family, and the little church that met in her house. Then it was my turn to pray. At these times in her tiny room, God was very near to us both. When I left, she always went with me to the gate. "Thank you for coming," she said. "Go in peace."

On hearing she was failing rapidly, I went at once to see her.

She was lying on her quilt on the hot floor. She took my hand.

"It's good to see you," she said, "but you needn't come again, for I won't be here. I'm going to meet my Savior and my children. If only my son were a Christian, I'd die happy. God has been good to me. Please pray," she whispered.

I prayed, but she had exhausted her strength and her breath, and her prayer was a silent one. Tearfully, for I knew I shouldn't see her again, I slipped away.

She died peacefully that night.

The next evening a carload from the hospital accompanied me to the usual worship service held at the placing of the body in the coffin. The scapegrace son wasn't there, but the daughter-in-law, grandchildren, Christians, and other neighbors attended. After singing a hymn of hope, Elder Lee thanked God for the good life now passed on, and asked for comfort and blessing on the family. When the wasted body, tinier than ever, was placed in the coffin I saw it was dressed in coarse homespun cotton.

"Why isn't she wearing the beautiful white-silk burial clothes she made for herself?" I asked in amazement. "She showed them to me a long time ago and told me she wanted to be buried in them."

The daughter-in-law hung her head and said nothing.

A neighbor replied. "She made those over for the children two or three years ago." How like her!

Burials are held on the third, fifth, or seventh day after the death. On the third day, I went to the funeral. Many were present, including the son. It would have been a scandal if he had not attended his mother's funeral. Elder Lee conducted the service with words of thanksgiving, comfort, and hope. Instead of the wailing for the dead, there was a hymn of praise and confidence.

Then the coffin was carried out to a grave dug at the foot of the hill behind the house.

"Is she to be buried here?" I asked in astonishment. "She told me herself she bought a burial site at the top of the hill and wanted to be buried there. She said all arrangements were made. Is her wish to be ignored?"

A neighbor helping carry the coffin shrugged his shoulders.

"Her son says it's too much trouble to carry the coffin up there."

So Grandmother Kang's tired body was laid to rest in the backyard, instead of the beautiful spot where she wished to lie. Her memory is blessed by all who knew her, and who can say she has not seen the children she lost so long ago?

-20-

The political situation was growing more and more difficult. Foreigners were watched, followed, and Koreans seen talking to foreigners were often called to the police station and questioned at length or detained overnight. Missionaries had to stop visiting country churches because such visits brought trouble for the local Christians.

Japanese orders to attend Shinto shrines and bow to the east, the direction of the Emperor's palace in Tokyo, were a matter of great heart burning to many, missionaries and Korean Christians alike.

The Federal Council of Missionaries asked the government authorities for an official statement as to whether this was a religious or a patriotic ceremony. They replied that it was not religious, but wholly patriotic, no more religious than placing flowers at a grave or saluting the flag as in Western countries. This being so, they said that everyone must comply and orders must be obeyed.

This explanation did not satisfy everybody. If attending the shrine and bowing were only a mark of respect to the Emperor, no one need object, but on the instructions to schools to attend the shrine ceremonies the character for worship was used. Some missionaries feared that even if they accepted the official statement, their attendance would make it more difficult for those whose consciences told them to refrain from attending.

People considered the matter from various angles. If the principal and teachers, as well as pupils, did not go to the shrine ceremonies, schools were likely to be closed and the principal punished. Thus, many children would be deprived of an education, the responsibility for which was a heavy load to bear.

Some Christian schools—both mission and church—rather than refuse to go and be forcibly closed, chose instead to close voluntarily. Others thought it would be better to attend the shrine and keep the schools open. Even those attending, Christian or not, certainly did not worship the Japanese Emperor. Christians, even at a shrine, prayed to God alone. Others felt that their presence would indicate they were worshiping the Japanese God-Emperor.

Whether shrine attendance was religious or patriotic was a real problem to many. Numbers of schools closed voluntarily to avoid shrine attendance or involuntarily as punishment for not doing so.

Those who refused to go and suffered in consequence sometimes were bitter at people taking the opposite attitude. They felt that if all Christians had agreed to do the same thing it would have been easier, since the compliance of some made it more difficult for the others.

Soon after World War II broke out in Europe in 1939, foreign embassies in Korea began advising their citizens to leave Korea. Not many passenger ships called there and, though families began to leave quite soon, it took a year or so for all to get away.

Meantime, the war in China continued to spread and no one knew whether the war in Europe or the one in China would most affect this part of the world.

When the first house in our small mission community became vacant when one of the families was recalled to Canada during the Depression, the mission agreed for the hospital to take it over. It was soon transformed into a medical annex with twenty beds. When a second house was vacated in the general evacuation of foreigners, the hospital took that over too, partly because of the need for more hospital beds and partly to forestall the authorities from occupying the house. We converted this second house, a fine stone building originally built by the Y M C A for one of their families, into a maternity annex under Dr. Kim Hyo-Soon, now an experienced staff doctor. This brought the number of hospital beds to one hundred, ten times what it was when I opened the hospital nearly twenty years before.

In Hamheung and other towns along the railway, every school had to send at least one class to the railway station to "comfort" the soldiers each time a troop train with Japanese soldiers went through on its way north. Even at five o'clock in the morning, long before daylight on cold winter days, small school children had to be on the platform. Since troop trains sometimes went through several times a day, this interfered considerably with schoolwork.

As a matter of economy, to help the war efforts of the country, people were ordered not to wear white, the traditional color of clothing in Korea. Most farmers and many other poor folk had no other clothes but white cotton. People coming to town to sell their farm produce entered the city by way of the bridge. To discourage wearing of white, a policeman was stationed with a pot of black paint and a large paintbrush to put blotches of black paint on the white clothes of those passing by. It was a common sight to see people with large black patches on their white clothing. Such senseless actions did little to promote patriotism for Japan in the Korean people, and it was difficult to see how it helped the economy.

At prayers one morning in the hospital, the leader for the day announced that we would sing several hymns instead of the usual one since this would be the last time we could sing them. The Japanese authorities had ordered that all hymns with the word Lord or King be torn out of the hymn books. If not, the books would be confiscated.

It was necessary to get police permission for any meeting except the regular church services. Such permission was rarely granted. In order to secure it, the group had to state the object of the meeting, name the speakers, and have their addresses approved by the police. Police were present at all public gatherings and, if they didn't like what was said, they interrupted the speaker who was likely to be taken to the police station or to prison. Spies were planted in every school, factory, church, and institution of every kind.

One old retired minister, the father of Dr. Lee of our Ear, Nose, and Throat Department, was asked to preach in a church without a pastor. During his sermon he told of seeing a wretched beggar on the street. The pastor wondered what was the cause of a person being in such a state of poverty. Was the man himself entirely to blame or was some of the responsibility for such a state of affairs on society? For this criticism of the regime the old man was imprisoned for many months.

About this time, two Japanese officials called on me one day and asked for a contribution to the army. That was one contribution I was determined not to make. I thought fast and told them that as a Christian I couldn't approve of the suffering, destruction, and loss of life caused by war. I believed in peace and couldn't make a contribution to the army, but to show my goodwill, if they sent around a collector for the Red Cross, I would be glad to make a generous contribution. They accepted this explanation and left without any sign of annoyance. I heard later that a missionary friend who had been outspoken enough against the Japanese to get himself into their bad graces, when asked, didn't dare refuse a contribution for the army.

In the midst of mounting tension, advised to go or ordered out by embassy officials, Ethel McEachren, Edna McLellan, and Ada Sandell left for Canada. Beulah Bourns, one of our nurses from a northern station, who had once before substituted for Ada when she was on furlough, came to live with me in our half empty house to take Ada's place in the hospital. With her came her assistant, Nurse Song Maria. The training of nurses and the supervision of the two annexes, as well as the main hospital and the tuberculosis building, kept Ada and Nurse Song busy.

Since people were now afraid to visit us freely as they had, committee rooms and guest rooms in our house were no longer needed. To conserve the scarce fuel, we closed half the house. A few loyal friends came quietly once in a while after dark, and it was good to see them. We got a small dog, named Minus because his tail had been cut short, and a kitten for company and amusement. Dogs are seldom pets in Korea and it was funny to see how devoted Jung-Ine our housekeeper became to the little dog. She would try to tuck him in his box behind the stove for the night before slipping away herself. But he would invariably jump out and go with her to the door. Then she went back and tucked him in again. This performance was generally repeated three or four times till one or the other won out.

Dr. Kim Hyo-Soon, woman staff member, had difficulty finding suitable quarters near the hospital, so we invited her to live with us. That suited her and we were glad to have another person in our half empty house.

About this time, an edict was issued that all Koreans, being Japanese subjects, must take Japanese names. They couldn't even choose their own, but must accept what was bestowed upon them. They hated losing their ancestral clan names by which a person could recognize his fellow clansmen wherever he met them. Members of the same clan were now given different names so they could no longer recognize one another. This was deeply resented. Of all the "patriotic" actions of the Japanese, this upset the Koreans more than anything else. Some wept as they told me their new names. Dr. Koh became Dr. Takahashi, a name he detested. Of course, we didn't use the Japanese names among ourselves, but they were now the legal ones and had to be used as signatures and on all legal documents.

Friends came to see us at the hospital instead of at our house. We understood. Some of them said they hoped we would stay with them throughout the hard times ahead if we felt we could take it.

By now, all our mission group had returned to Canada except Mr. Scott, Beulah Bourns, and myself in Hamheung, and Mr. Fraser in Wonsan. Wonsan with its beautiful sheltered harbor, said to be one of the six best in the world, was a big Japanese naval base. Since the Fraser home was on a hilltop overlooking the harbor, it would not have been wise for any foreigner to try to remain there at that time. He would certainly be arrested as a spy. But if Mr. Fraser were in any trouble, he couldn't communicate with the rest of us. He could hardly expect to remain in freedom if and when Japan entered the World War raging in Europe. We persuaded him to move to Hamheung where our group would at least be together in the same city. He and Mr. Scott lived in the Scott house just over the hill from ours.

Amidst mounting pressure and almost complete curtailment of mission work other than the medical and the schools, it was urgent to plan how best to carry on—or to decide if carrying on was the wisest course.

Mission property left unoccupied would be considered abandoned and taken over by the government. If turned over to the Korean church or any board or foundation (the formation of which would likely be forbidden, or at least permission refused), the members could be intimitated or the property confiscated. Partly to try to hold the property for future use by the mission and partly to share with Korean friends the hard times they were enduring, Mr. Fraser and Mr. Scott decided to stay as long as possible. Beulah and I felt since we were women, and as such didn't count for much in Japanese eyes, we might be permitted to continue the medical work. The two men agreed and our board in Canada gave its consent.

How long would we be able to continue? Where and how could we get supplies? How could we manage if and when mission funds could not reach us? If the war in China spread to Korea, hospitals would be needed more than ever. Under such conditions, we thought the medical work would likely be allowed to continue. We considered that though I as a foreigner probably would not be allowed to continue as superintendent, Dr. Koh—now Dr. Takahashi—as a Japanese subject probably could. He might, of course, be replaced by a Japanese, but we could only take a chance on that.

We suggested to the hospital board, most of whom were Koreans, that Dr. Koh would have a better chance to carry on than I. They agreed and he was asked to return to Hamheung as superintendent. He returned to take over, though not able at once to relinquish all his responsibilities at Severance.

The church people decided to have a celebration recognizing my twenty years in Korea and Dr. Koh's becoming superintendent. Many of the public including some officials attended the gathering and several speeches of encouragement for him and appreciation of my work were given. Under Dr. Koh as superintendent, I continued as head of the maternity, gynecology, and tuberculosis departments.

In July 1941, we four foreigners went to Whajinpo Beach where many Westerners had summer cottages. The Japanese had moved us off Wonsan Beach a few years earlier. We went to check the condition of the summer cottages on the beach and what, if anything, could be done to protect them. It was rather lonely seeing this deserted place where we had so often met with friends, most of whom were no longer in Korea.

Day after day, from morning till night, we saw ships going north, loaded, we supposed, with Japanese troops and war supplies. The war in China was still raging and now it looked as if something bigger were afoot. We heard later that this movement of troops was to take part in a clash with Russia somewhere along the border, in which Japan lost heavily.

On the fourth day of our stay at the beach, an urgent message came from Hamheung. We must return at once and report to the authorities within forty-eight hours the exact amount of money we had. All foreign funds were to be frozen.

At the railway station, only two tickets were available. The men wouldn't let us stay behind alone so we went ahead with Edith Myers, a nurse from Pyungyang who had already had her ticket. She was to accompany us as far north as Wonsan where she expected to get a cross-country train direct to Pyungyang. Some Roman Catholic priests from that city, finding they couldn't get tickets, started to walk overland. Our two mission men were to come next day when two more tickets would be available.

Edith had never been in Wonsan; she didn't know the city or where the Fraser house was where she was to spend the night. So Beulah went with her. From the train I saw them both taken to the police station. What did that mean? Should I go and join them or might I be able to do more for them by staying out of trouble? As the train began to move, they clambered breathlessly on board.

"The police won't let us stay in Wonsan," they said. "They demanded to know what we were doing here, said we had no permission to come to Wonsan, and must get out at once. 'Get out! Get out!' they shouted at us."

At Hamheung, we were all ordered into the police station. Two women had left here and three had come back. Who was the stranger and why hadn't she a ticket for Hamheung?

We explained the circumstances. The outside man, who had met us, now spoke up for us and was struck over the head for it. Meanwhile one of the policemen was phoning Wonsan for confirmation of our story. When this was forthcoming they let us go with what we, perhaps rather unjustly, felt was real reluctance.

Next morning, I accompanied Edith Myers to the station to see, if I could, that she got on the train. She decided to go to Seoul and north from there up the west coast instead of trying to change trains at Wonsan. Since I wasn't allowed on the platform, I joined a group of Korean women who had come to see someone off and weren't allowed outside the wicket either. Several Japanese soldiers without a word of warning made at us with fixed bayonets. We took the hint and left the station. I stayed as near as I could to take Edith back with me if she couldn't get on the train. I heard it pull out and when she didn't return, I hoped she was on her way. A letter some days later told us she had reached home without further adventure.

The two men arrived the day after we did and the necessary reports were made within the deadline. In order to be ready for any eventualities, we had all been saving up to have something on hand when supplies should be shut off. Mission and all foreign owned funds were frozen, but we had permission to draw living expenses and wages for those working for us.

In October 1941, Mr. Scott and Mr. Fraser, with the British consul's permission, went to Yongjung to make a contract with the Japanese army for use of the mission residences that they were about to take over. The men told us to expect them back in about five days, and if they encountered any difficulties that would delay them, they would let us know.

When five days went by without any word and they hadn't returned, we began to fear they were in some sort of trouble, but there was nothing we could do about it. There was no possibility of communicating with them since we didn't know where they were. As days went by, our concern increased. Had they been taken into custody? Why was there no word from them?

Finally, I went to see Elder Lee of the Y M C A, a trusted friend and advisor, and told him the circumstances as far as we knew them. Should we do something, I asked him, and if so, what? Would it be wise to inform the British Embassy that the two who had gone to Manchuria hadn't returned? Since all our letters were censored, would such a letter be delivered?

Elder Lee was reassuring. He counseled waiting another day or two instead of doing anything hastily. This turned out to be the wise advice for the missing men returned a couple of days later.

On December 7, 1941, Beulah and I were at the hospital as usual and Mr. Scott was teaching at the Yungsaing Boys' Academy when a Korean gendarme came to see me.

"The Japanese have attacked Pearl Harbor," he said, "and outside of the gendarmerie you're the first in the city to know it. That means war, but don't be afraid. You'll be safe here. We'll take care of you. Don't let anyone know I told you." He slipped away. I found Beulah and told her.

The gendarme then informed Mr. Fraser at the Scott house.

Mr. Scott, on his way home from the academy, dropped in at the hospital and I told him what I'd heard. Thus, we were all prepared to meet the Japanese gendarmes who came a little later to inform us we were enemy aliens. We showed no surprise.

"You needn't be afraid," they too told us. "We'll protect you."

We didn't feel any need of protection from Koreans, but weren't so sure of the Japanese. We didn't know how much of what they said was really meant.

"Now let us go to your house," they said. "Take your coats with you."

When the staff saw us leave the hospital wearing our winter overcoats and accompanied by Japanese military police, they were much distressed, fearing we were under arrest and being taken away to internment—perhaps imprisonment.

"If anyone annoys you," the gendarmes told us, "just report it to us and we'll see it doesn't happen again. You two women may continue to live in this house, but you mustn't go anywhere else. You must understand that."

"That means," I said, "that we can't go in the streets, to the market, and to church, but what about the hospital? Can't we do our usual work there?"

"You may go to the hospital as usual, but remember, nowhere else."

Beulah and I looked at one another. It might have been much worse, and if we could continue to carry on our work our staying in Korea would be worthwhile. In a sense, it was an adventure. It certainly was a new experience and we felt exhilarated.

"Now," went on the military man, "bring me your radio and cameras. I have to seal them up. I'll need lots of old newspapers too."

He wrapped and tied up our cameras and radio in many layers of newspapers, sealed them in several places with a seal, and left them with us, with the warning that the seals must, on no account, be broken. Then, saying he would look in on us from time to time, he left.

Two gendarmes remained on guard at the men's house. That evening others came to say they would have to detain Mr. Fraser in the gendarmerie because of what they thought was "complicity in the spying activities of an Englishman working for an oil storage company near Wonsan." He was allowed to take his overcoat and a blanket or two.

The guards watched Mr. Scott eat, accompanied him to the bathroom, and remained in his room as he slept. What was happening to Mr. Fraser we didn't know but, knowing that many people who had the misfortune to be taken to the gendarmerie were tortured, we feared the worst. We heard about Mr. Fraser through the cook at the men's house, who told our cook, who told us. We were not allowed any direct communication with the other foreigners. From the hill behind our house, I once waved toward the other home, but was firmly told that could not be permitted.

Dr. Kim Hyo-Soon felt it would be wiser for her to leave our house where she would likely be under suspicion, and she moved out. One cold night, her landlady told a child to put a hot-water bottle—a big crockery affair known as a pig—in her bed. The doctor was kept late at the hospital by a maternity case and when she finally climbed into her bed, the carelessly placed bottle had overturned and there was ice on her sheets.

Sometime in the night I was awakened by something very cold getting into bed with me. Dr. Kim still had our door key. I got her warmed up and from then on she came every night sometime after dark. Song Maria came too and slept with Beulah. They did this so we would not be alone. It was good of them, and they took considerable risk to do it. They knew perfectly well that the military police often chose the middle of the night to make surprise raids on people they were interested in, and it would likely go hard with anyone found in our house.

One day Beulah, in great excitement, told me of a young German woman who was being admitted to the hospital. Beulah had offered to take her two small children into our house and look after them while their mother was sick. Beulah loved children and this was a happy task for her. The father wanted to rent our house, she added. "We've lots of room, so we might as well, don't you think?"

"Germans!" I exclaimed. "What are Germans doing here? There never were any before. We've got to remember we're now enemy aliens on the other side from the Germans in the war. No doubt they'd like to have our house to live in, and think how convenient it would be to spy on us."

"I never thought of that," said Beulah, who never suspected anyone of evil intentions. "Anyway, we'll have to look after the children. They can't make any trouble for us, and as long as they're here we can't keep their father away, can we?"

"I suppose not, but let's not encourage him to come or to rent the house. After all, it's not ours. It belongs to the mission and we just can't do anything we like with it. What is that fellow doing here anyway?"

"He works at the big fertilizer factory at Heungnam."

"That may explain a lot." There was indeed a fertilizer factory, but it was always kept so hush-hush that no one working there was allowed in any section except the one he worked in. No visitors were ever permitted. We had long suspected that war supplies were also manufactured there as well as fertilizer. Likely enough, the man wanted to spy on us. When I met the big arrogant fellow I wasn't at all reassured.

When the mother recovered, the family went back to

Heungnam, and the lonely woman who could talk to no one but her husband called on us occasionally.

With no home letters, no guests, and no going to church, Christmas was a lonely occasion. After rounds in the hospital, when the others went off to church, rather than return to our dreary house, we walked around in the snow in the hospital grounds until we got thoroughly chilled.

We had hardly got in when the cook from the Scott house arrived to tell us we were invited to Christmas dinner.

"What's that?" I asked, incredulous. "You know we aren't allowed to go there."

"Yes, you are. The gendarme said you might come."

"You're sure?"

"Yes. He said you might come today to dinner."

"Does Mr. Scott know? Is he expecting us?"

"He knows. He sent me to tell you. He wasn't allowed to write a note."

"When was this decided? Is there dinner enough for us too?"

"Well, perhaps you better bring your dinner with you."

Carrying our dinner we knocked on the Scott door wondering who would open it, the man of the house—if he were still man of the house—or one of the guards. Mr. Scott himself, looking rather subdued, opened it and greeted us quietly in English.

"Merry Christmas," said he. "I'm going to get in a few words in our own language since I don't know how long we'll be allowed to speak it. Come in. Come in. It's good to see you."

Three guards were sitting around the living room, their rifles leaning up in a corner. While we were wondering how we should greet them, they relieved our embarrassment by speaking politely to us first.

With three guards behind our chairs, three rifles in the corner, not knowing how much we might be allowed to say, or what might be happening to Mr. Fraser, it was not a very festive Christmas dinner. This was specially so since the guards, had told Mr. Scott that Mr. Fraser would be home before Christmas. When he hadn't come, we feared some complication. Mr. Scott shared dinner with the guards, who no doubt would have preferred their own food, but were interested in tasting ours. When one of them demanded to know what Christmas was and why it was celebrated, Mr. Scott explained.

After we finished eating, our host told us he had permission to read the Christmas story and to pray in our own language, but if he wanted to preach or give a talk it would have to be in Korean. He would read and pray only. He prayed at considerable length, informing the Almighty of various circumstances undoubtedly known to Him, but enlightening to us. He thanked the Lord that "our brother," mentioning no names, was comfortable as he had been permitted a small stove in his cell, that he was allowed to have his food sent to him from this house, that he had his overcoat and a couple of blankets with him, and that he hadn't been subjected to any physical hardship. He thanked God that investigation hadn't found any evidence of wrongdoing and that there was hope our brother would soon be permitted to return home. Mr. Scott also expressed gratitude for various other things and circumstances and made petition for peace, goodwill, and justice on the earth. When the prayer was interrupted with demands to interpret what had been said, there was enough to put into Korean that it wasn't obvious some was omitted.

We went home with lighter hearts than when we had come, but that Christmas evening we heard that Hong Kong, where Canadian troops had recently arrived, had fallen, a blow we expected, but not anticipated quite so soon.

One day Mr. Scott happened to glance up at a high shelf in his study and was horrified to see a small camera left by one of his boys. Possession of an undeclared camera could be considered a grave offense. How could he dispose of it without being seen? One day the guard coming on duty was late and the one to go off became impatient. He ordered Mr.

Scott to go outside while he went to the next house to phone. Our phones had been disconnected. Saying he was cold, Mr. Scott asked permission to go in the house to get a coat and before the guard got back he secured the camera, wrenched the lens out of it, and thrust it in a hole in the wall.

Soon after Christmas, Mr. Fraser was released. The guards left the Scott house and we were permitted to visit back and forth between the two houses. Thereafter, the guards did not too frequently visit both places. On New Year's Day, the four of us had dinner together without guards, a more cheerful occasion than Christmas with Mr. Fraser in detention.

Once a month, one letter from our home folks was doled out to us, letters that had come before communications were cut off but withheld from us then. Each time we got one, we thought it would be the last, but a month later one more was handed over. Old as they were, they were a link with home and it was good to get them. We wondered how many of our letters had got through to Canada during the last weeks before we were interned.

It was hard to read the papers in those times. The only ones we could read were English papers published in Japan. They described how the cowardly Americans in the Philippines put Filipino women and children in the front lines as hostages while they themselves sat comfortably and safely in deep trenches in the rear. They told of the brutal British in Hong Kong and Singapore who placed Chinese and Malay women and children out in front of their lines to face the brunt of the danger while they stayed in relative safety in the rear. They gave accounts of the terrible torture inflicted on any unfortunate Japanese soldiers stoutly defending the homeland, when any of them fell into the hands of the treacherous enemy.

"Dr. Koh," I asked one day after reading these accounts in the papers, "do people believe these horrible stories about British and American soldiers?"

"Of course anybody who knows any Western people realizes such stories can't be true," he replied, "but how many of our people have ever met a Western foreigner?"

Although all our radios were supposed to be sealed up, there was one that had been left behind by someone who had gone. It was only a six-tube radio, but an exceptionally good one. When the guards sealed up the four we owned, they didn't ask if there were others. Whether this one was left out by accident or design I don't know, but I like to give our friendly guards who treated us as well as they dared the benefit of the doubt.

After the guards left the Scott house and we had permission to visit, we often went in the evenings to listen to the radio news. While one of the men walked around outside to give the alarm if anyone approached, we others went upstairs where the radio was hidden. We placed it in the middle of a double bed with the mattress underneath and quilts over it to deaden the sound. We would uncover only enough of the front to let the sound out, put our heads close, and turn it up just enough for us to hear. When the British station went off the air at the fall of Hong Kong, we used to listen to an English broadcast from the French station that was able to continue for a while longer. We sometimes heard another station broadcasting in English from somewhere in China.

The two men were not allowed other visitors, even if any had been bold enough to venture to go to see them. On a few occasions when the Japanese gendarme was annoyed over something and in a bad temper he would forbid them to come to our house for a few days. Then one of the Korean guards would give permission again. At the hospital anyone could come and see Beulah and me, give us any news they had, and we passed it on to the men.

Our faithful housekeeper Jung-Ine looked after us as best she could. We always had plenty to eat, such as it was. Friends sometimes sent in a whole cooked dinner with the wish that we could come and eat it with them at their house, but since that was impossible, we should please eat it and think of them. Our food was as good and as plentiful as anyone else had, and what more could we expect? We missed bread and butter the most I think. We hadn't had bread for six months and butter for a year. One day Whang Changno, father of Dr. Whang who cared for Miss Robb when she fractured her leg, sent us a whole fresh salmon. Nothing ever tasted better.

So the winter went by and spring came again with its balmy breezes, green leaves, and flowers, while war ravaged more and more of the world. We didn't know how much of what we were allowed to hear was true.

When the Doolittle raid over Japan was announced, the papers reported eight American planes shot down over Japan. A day or two later, it was announced that one of the eight was to be exhibited all over the Japanese empire. Koreans said at once, "Eight planes were shot down and only one is to be exhibited? Ha, only one was shot down." We learned later that none were lost over Japan.

About this time our guards told us that we would be repatriated before long, but that we must each first write a statement on what we thought about the war and how it was likely to end. This caused some hard thinking. If we wrote anything not agreeable to the authorities, we might not be repatriated. On the other hand, we could hardly bring ourselves to say that we thought Japan was in the right or wanted her to win.

I wrote that since war resulted in such suffering, loss, and destruction of property and human life, I hoped it would be brought to an end as speedily as possible. I wanted to see justice done and therefore wished that whichever side was in the right would win. This was accepted.

In April our guards told us we were soon to be exchanged for Japanese coming from the United States and Canada, and we were to pack up and be ready to leave within a few days. We must hand over three copies of a list of the things we were leaving behind. All we could take, they told us, was what we could personally carry. No books, pictures, maps, nor printed matter could be taken with us. Even the maps in our Bibles would have to be torn out if we wanted to take the Bibles. After we had packed our trunks, they told us to unpack and make eleven copies of the list of articles in the trunks, including such trifles as pencils or hairpins. I tried to give some things away to friends, but was afraid to give much to any one person or anything readily identifiable as foreign, lest it might bring trouble to the person receiving it.

When our friends heard we were to leave, they were much concerned. Would we really be allowed to return to our country or be taken to an internment camp somewhere?

"How long do you think this war will last?" asked the furnace man. "When can you come back to Korea?"

"Who can predict that? It may take five years for the Allies to win," I said.

"Aren't the Japanese and Germans winning? All the papers tell of their winning victory after victory."

"It seems like that now, but you must remember they planned and prepared for war. Our people didn't plan nor prepare for it. It takes time to produce war materials and to train soldiers."

"What if," he persisted reasonably enough, "what if while the Allies are preparing, the Axis wins?"

"I don't know how long it will take for the Allies to catch up with the Japanese, Germans, and Italians, I don't know what may happen in the meantime, but I do know the spirit of my people. However long it takes, they'll never stop till they win. We'll be back all right."

Who could have foreseen that Roosevelt and Stalin, who together overruled Churchill at the Yalta Conference, would deliver half of Korea—unbeknownst to Koreans—into the hands of Russian communism?

After all was packed the second time, a delay of several weeks occurred during negotiations in Tokyo and we had to unpack in order to carry on the business of living. Departure was merely postponed they told us, not canceled, but for how long we had no idea, and no means of knowing if this were true or not.

A few weeks later, they told us we were to leave on the first of June, 1942, and they were going to allow us to have a farewell party to which all our friends could come without fear of consequences. This seemed almost too good to be true, but so it proved.

A Korean policeman who had replaced the gendarmes had all along been as lenient as he dared. He was the guard on duty at the party. He went at once into the farthest corner of the room and appeared to go asleep until it was time for the affair to break up. It was good to see friends we hadn't seen in six months and sad to think we might not see them again for years, if ever. There was plenty of talk, but none of the usual fun of a party. Before it broke up, several of the elders and our two mission men led in earnest prayer.

Next morning the same policeman escorted us, carrying our two suitcases each to the railway station. He walked in front of us and never once looked back to see who might be greeting us.

As we passed the hospital gate the whole staff, employees, and as many of the patients as could leave their beds were at the gate to wave goodbye. They didn't dare accompany us to the railway station, but tears flowed as we bade each other farewell. No one knew when we might meet again or what might befall any of us. They feared we were being taken away to be imprisoned and we knew hard times were in store for them.

At the station we saw Dr. Ahn, my first language teacher and his family, and Elder Kim Neung Keun, Mr. Scott's successor as principal of the boys' academy and we knew they were there as friends, though neither we nor they ventured to speak.

Once aboard the southbound train we watched, eyes dim with tears, as the familiar landscape slid away, slowly, then more rapidly, until Dragon Hill faded into the distance.